AF787042

Epizootics - Outbreaks of Animal Disease

Edited by David M. Claborn

Published in London, United Kingdom

Epizootics - Outbreaks of Animal Disease
http://dx.doi.org/10.5772/intechopen.1003308
Edited by David M. Claborn

Contributors
Adis Softić, Adriana Amfim, Afagh Torkan, Berhan Tamir, Binu T. Velayudhan, Cristina Jurado-Díaz, David M. Claborn, Ermin Šaljić, Jasmin Omeragić, Livia Cătălina Bercea, Mahdi Askari Badouei, Meera Surendran-Nair, Naida Kapo, Natalia Cucu, Olivia Sinn Kay Chan, Sandra Barroso-Arévalo, Shaun van den Hurk, Tefera Yilma, Teufik Goletić, Tewodros Eshete, Tilaye Demisse, Tommy TY Lam, Vedad Škapur, Šejla Goletić

© The Editor(s) and the Author(s) 2025
The rights of the editor(s) and the author(s) have been asserted in accordance with the Copyright, Designs and Patents Act 1988. All rights to the book as a whole are reserved by INTECHOPEN LIMITED. The book as a whole (compilation) cannot be reproduced, distributed or used for commercial or non-commercial purposes without INTECHOPEN LIMITED's written permission. Enquiries concerning the use of the book should be directed to INTECHOPEN LIMITED rights and permissions department (permissions@intechopen.com).
Violations are liable to prosecution under the governing Copyright Law.

Individual chapters of this publication are distributed under the terms of the Creative Commons Attribution 4.0 License which permits commercial use, distribution and reproduction of the individual chapters, provided the original author(s) and source publication are appropriately acknowledged. If so indicated, certain images may not be included under the Creative Commons license. In such cases users will need to obtain permission from the license holder to reproduce the material. More details and guidelines concerning content reuse and adaptation can be found at http://www.intechopen.com/copyright-policy.html.

Notice
Statements and opinions expressed in the chapters are these of the individual contributors and not necessarily those of the editors or publisher. No responsibility is accepted for the accuracy of information contained in the published chapters. The publisher assumes no responsibility for any damage or injury to persons or property arising out of the use of any materials, instructions, methods or ideas contained in the book.

First published in London, United Kingdom, 2025 by IntechOpen
IntechOpen is the global imprint of INTECHOPEN LIMITED, registered in England and Wales, registration number: 11086078, 167-169 Great Portland Street, London, W1W 5PF, United Kingdom

For EU product safety concerns: IN TECH d.o.o., Prolaz Marije Krucifikse Kozulić 3, 51000 Rijeka, Croatia, info@intechopen.com or visit our website at intechopen.com.

British Library Cataloguing-in-Publication Data
A catalogue record for this book is available from the British Library

Epizootics - Outbreaks of Animal Disease
Edited by David M. Claborn
p. cm.

This title is part of the Veterinary Medicine and Science Book Series, Volume 22
Topic: Animal Science
Series Editor: Rita Payan Carreira
Topic Editor: Edward Narayan

Print ISBN 978-0-85014-894-7
Online ISBN 978-0-85014-893-0
eBook (PDF) ISBN 978-0-85014-895-4
ISSN 2632-0517

If disposing of this product, please recycle the paper responsibly.

We are IntechOpen, the world's leading publisher of Open Access books

Built by scientists, for scientists

7,300+
Open access books available

193,000+
International authors and editors

210M+
Downloads

156
Countries delivered to

Our authors are among the
Top 1%
most cited scientists

12.2%
Contributors from top 500 universities

WEB OF SCIENCE™

Selection of our books indexed in the Book Citation Index
in Web of Science™ Core Collection (BKCI)

Interested in publishing with us?
Contact book.department@intechopen.com

Numbers displayed above are based on latest data collected.
For more information visit www.intechopen.com

IntechOpen Book Series

Veterinary Medicine and Science

Volume 22

Aims and Scope of the Series

Paralleling similar advances in the medical field, astounding advances occurred in Veterinary Medicine and Science in recent decades. These advances have helped foster better support for animal health, more humane animal production, and a better understanding of the physiology of endangered species to improve the assisted reproductive technologies or the pathogenesis of certain diseases, where animals can be used as models for human diseases (like cancer, degenerative diseases or fertility), and even as a guarantee of public health. Bridging Human, Animal, and Environmental health, the holistic and integrative "One Health" concept intimately associates the developments within those fields, projecting its advancements into practice. This book series aims to tackle various animal-related medicine and sciences fields, providing thematic volumes consisting of high-quality significant research directed to researchers and postgraduates. It aims to give us a glimpse into the new accomplishments in the Veterinary Medicine and Science field. By addressing hot topics in veterinary sciences, we aim to gather authoritative texts within each issue of this series, providing in-depth overviews and analysis for graduates, academics, and practitioners and foreseeing a deeper understanding of the subject. Forthcoming texts, written and edited by experienced researchers from both industry and academia, will also discuss scientific challenges faced today in Veterinary Medicine and Science. In brief, we hope that books in this series will provide accessible references for those interested or working in this field and encourage learning in a range of different topics.

Meet the Series Editor

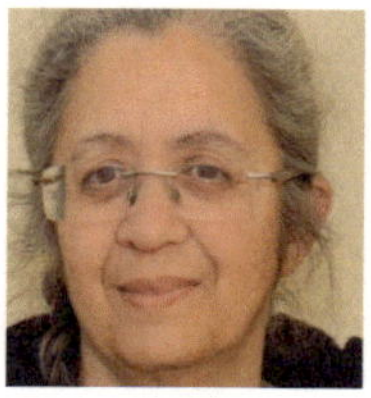

Rita Payan Carreira earned her Veterinary Degree from the Faculty of Veterinary Medicine in Lisbon, Portugal, in 1985. She obtained her Ph.D. in Veterinary Sciences from the University of Trás-os-Montes e Alto Douro, Portugal. After almost 32 years of teaching at the University of Trás-os-Montes and Alto Douro, she recently moved to the University of Évora, Department of Veterinary Medicine, where she teaches in the field of Animal Reproduction and Clinics. Her primary research areas include the molecular markers of the endometrial cycle and the embryo–maternal interaction, including oxidative stress and the reproductive physiology and disorders of sexual development, besides the molecular determinants of male and female fertility. She often supervises students preparing their master's or doctoral theses. She is also a frequent referee for various journals.

Meet the Volume Editor

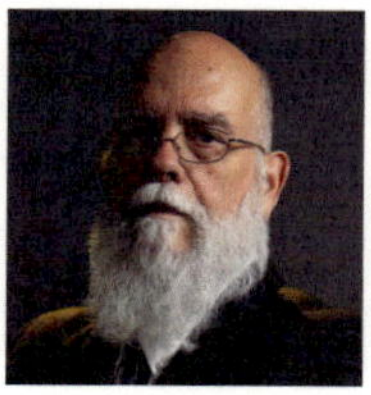

David Claborn started his professional career as a public health entomologist for the U.S. Navy, allowing him to work internationally. He has spent about eight years working outside the U.S., from Venezuela to South Korea. He was also stationed with the U.S. Marine Corps in Saudi Arabia during Operation Desert Storm. He completed his Doctor of Public Health (DrPH) degree at the Uniformed Services University of the Health Sciences in 2001. After retiring from the Navy at the rank of Commander in 2008, he moved to Missouri State University, where he served as the director of the Master of Public Health program for 10 years. In 2023, he became the Associate Dean of the College of Healthcare Technologies at the American University of Iraq-Baghdad.

Contents

Preface

Just like human populations, animal populations may experience significant outbreaks of disease. In humans, these outbreaks may be referred to as "epidemics" or, if they cover large geographic areas, "pandemics". The term "epidemic" may not be sufficiently accurate for animal populations because the base upon which the word is built ",-deme", means people. Therefore, the word "epizootic" is often preferred when referring to disease outbreaks in animal populations.

Epizootics can be devastating to animal populations, even resulting in extinction in some cases. It is worth noting that the same can happen in plants, as demonstrated by the American Chestnut blight; however, recent epizootics of fungal diseases in frogs and bats demonstrate the potential for rapid die-offs in animals. Some epizootics, like that caused by the West Nile virus, which has killed millions of birds, may also cause epidemics in human populations, but the importance of epizootics is not limited to their effects on humans.

Although several categories of disease cause epizootics, with agents ranging from fungal to viral, one category that has had great importance in recent years is that of vector-borne diseases. This emphasis is reflected in this book. Some authorities have linked recent vector-borne disease outbreaks to climate change. However, others will point toward other issues such as reduced vector control efforts, environmental changes like deforestation or reforestation, resurgence of deer populations, and introduction of invasive species. These factors can contribute to the importance of vector-borne diseases in animal populations.

The chapters in this book reflect current perspectives and changes in the causes and directions of disease outbreaks in animal populations. If recent developments in the field foretell upcoming outbreaks, there will be a need for several updates to this book.

David M. Claborn
College of Healthcare Technologies,
American University of Iraq-Baghdad,
Baghdad, Iraq

Section 1

Introduction

Chapter 1

Introductory Chapter: Epizootics as a Field of Study – The Importance Is Not Limited to Human Health

David M. Claborn

1.Introduction

An etymologist might say that the word "epidemiology" is based on three Greek words:
"epi-"meaning "on",
"demos" meaning "the people or country" and
"logos" meaning "knowledge or study".

There are other meanings for these words, especially "logos", but literally translated, "epidemiology" would mean "the study of that which is upon the people." Obviously, this is talking about disease that affects a human population, and there have been many such diseases, from pneumonic plague to COVID-19. But this anthropocentric perspective ignores the fact that animals also have their diseases, and many of them are shared with humans. In fact, the two diseases mentioned above had zoonotic origins, plague in rodents and COVID-19 mostly likely in bats. Sometimes disease outbreaks in animals move into the human population and when this happens, the disease is a zoonotic disease. For obvious reasons, these are the animal diseases that are of most interest to humans. However, animals also have their own "epidemics", and those diseases can be devastating to the animal population. Strictly speaking, these epidemics in animals should be called "epizootics."

2. Background

Three diseases provide good examples of just how much disease can affect an animal population: white-nose syndrome in bats, chytridiomycosis in amphibians, and West Nile virus in crows. This introduction will briefly describe these diseases because they have had significant effects on the animals which each infects, and they demonstrate how devastating epizootics can occur, often with little public attention. However, before describing these diseases and discussing why everyone should be interested in such diseases, it is helpful to realize the wide variety and geographic range of animal diseases. **Table 1** is a selection of diseases found in animal hosts over a brief period of one month and as reported in the disease reporting program ProMed, a service of the International Society for Infectious Diseases (Available from: http://www.promedmail.org). The table is a selection of the diseases reported and is not exhaustive. Note the wide range of diseases, hosts, and geographic regions listed in the table.

Disease or agent	Country	Animal affected	Date of report
Q fever	Montenegro	Livestock	12 Sep 24
Avian influenza	Israel	Poultry	18 Sep 24
Crimean-Congo Hemorrhagic fever	Israel	Cattle	18 Sep 24
Avian botulism	USA	Wild birds	16 Sep 24
New World Screwworm	Costa Rica	Sloth	24 Sep 24
Anthrax	El Salvador	Cattle	18 Sep 24
Rabies	USA	Bat	27 Sep 24
Rat Hepatitis C	USA	Pigs	25 Sep 24
Myxomytosis	Germany	Rabbits	21 Sep 24
Eastern Equine Encephalitis	USA	Horse	30 Sep 24
New World Screw Worm	Honduras	Cattle	18 Sep 24
Bovine Spongilliform Encephalopathy	Ireland	Cattle	3 Oct 24
Avian influenza	Japan	Wild birds	4 Oct 24
Epizootic hemorrhagic disease	USA	Deer	8 Oct 24
Glanders	India	Horses	8 Oct 24
Trichonellosis	USA	Bear	10 Oct 24
Blue tongue virus	Netherlands	Sheep, cattle	11 Oct 24
Lumpy Skin disease	Algeria	Cattle	12 Oct 24
African Swine fever	South Korea	Pigs	13 Oct 24

Table 1.
Selected outbreaks in animals during a period of one month (12 September to 13 October, 2024) as reported in the ProMed disease reporting system.

One disease has been described as the worst infectious disease to have occurred in vertebrate populations, based in part on its ability to drive species toward extinction and to affect numerous species [1]. This disease is unfamiliar to many people because it affects amphibians. It is caused by a fungus, providing the disease with the name "chytridiomycosis". Scientists have observed for many years that amphibian populations have been diminishing, but in the 1990's, a sudden decline occurred even in pristine environments. This observation suggested that the declines were not the result of human-caused pollution to the environment, so additional research was initiated to find the cause. Eventually, researchers found that the fungus *Batrachonchytrium dendobatides* was the likely cause of the population decline. Subsequent work suggests that multiple related fungal species are responsible for the worldwide decline. The fungus has driven many frog species into extinction and other species have suffered mass die-offs that have driven populations into permanent decline. The fungus appears to affect the skin in such a way that the frogs cannot regulate electrolytes, leading to death.

At the turn of the century, crows in the USA experienced a similar die-off. Though not driven to extinction, the large American crow population suffered enormous mortality and this was due to the recently introduced West Nile virus. This virus had been known in the Old World for quite a while but it was introduced to the USA in the summer of 1999. Early reports of the disease were associated with human cases, in part due to several cases of flaccid paralysis caused by the disease. With time, however, the virus was identified in bird populations. The mortality to the bird populations was so dramatic that the spread of the virus across the country could be roughly traced merely by counting the dead birds. The corvid population, including crows and jays, appeared to be especially vulnerable to the disease. One study using traced birds concluded that more than two-thirds of the American crows in Illinois died as a result of West Nile virus [2].

A final example of a catastrophic epizootic is provided by White-Nose syndrome in bats. This is, again, caused by a fungus. The infection seems to interrupt hibernation in the bats which depletes their fat reserves. Especially during long winters, the depleted fat stores lead to the death of the bats [3]. At least six species of bats have been infected resulting in "unprecedented deaths of hibernating bats". Laboratory studies suggest that for bats that are infected with this fungus, mortality ranges between 90 and 100% [4].

3. Conclusion

The two fungal diseases for bats and amphibians do not appear to be dangerous for humans; the West Nile virus, however, is an important human disease and is the vector-borne disease with the widest range, spanning much of the globe. The ecological effects of all of these diseases are more than significant, even when they do not have direct impacts on human health. Understanding these outbreaks and epizootics is essential; the importance extends well beyond that of direct impact on human health. The extinction of species, as has been seen with frogs, can have permanent effects on ecological balance. Even in the absence of related human disease, the study of epizootics is essential. Nevertheless, when the human disease factor is added, there is much more interest in the study of zoonotic disease.

One proposal to deal with the toll of zoonotic disease is the concept of One Health. This concept seeks to integrate the knowledge and skills from multiple disciplines, including human medicine, veterinary medicine, biology, ecology, engineering and others. The purpose of that collaboration is to address complex health challenges by utilization of diverse knowledge sources in a more complete understanding of the ways human health, animal health, the environment, and political realities interact to affect human health [5]. One Health is a concept that is usually based on improving human health, so it may ignore epizootics that have little impact on humans. Such blindness can be very harmful when disease agents emerge from an animal reservoir, as with the case of COVID-19. Nevertheless, epizootics with little or no direct effect on human health are important in themselves. Their impact on the environment may not be realized for decades, but many will be important for a long time.

Author details

David M. Claborn
College of Allied Health Sciences, American University of Iraq-Baghdad, Iraq

*Address all correspondence to: claborn@auib.edu.iq

IntechOpen

© 2024 The Author(s). Licensee IntechOpen. This chapter is distributed under the terms of the Creative Commons Attribution License (http://creativecommons.org/licenses/by/4.0), which permits unrestricted use, distribution, and reproduction in any medium, provided the original work is properly cited.

References

[1] Rooij V, Pascale AM, Haesebrouck F, Pasmans F. Amphibian chytridiomycosis: A review with focus on fungus-host interactions. Veterinary Research. 2015;**46**:137

[2] Yaremych RE, Warner PC, Mankin JD, Brawn AR, Novak R. West Nile virus and high death rate in American crows. Emerging Infectious Diseases. 2004;**10**:709-711

[3] Wibbelt G, Kurth A, Hellmann D, Weishaar M, Barlow A, Veith M, et al. White-nose syndrome fungus (*Geomyces destructans*) in bats, Europe. Emerging Infectious Diseases. 2010;**16**(8):1237-1242

[4] National Park Service (n.d.) What is White-Nose Syndrome? Available from: https://www.nps.gov/articles/what-is-white-nose-syndrome.htm

[5] Errecaborde KM, Macy KW, Pekol A, Perez S, O'Brien MK, Allen I. Factors that enable effective one health collaborations-a scoping review of the literature. PLoS One. 2019;**14**(12):e0224660. DOI: 10.1371/journal.pone.0224660

Chapter 2

Animal Disease Surveillance: History of Zoonotic Viruses and Bacteria and Diagnostics

Olivia Sinn Kay Chan, Meera Surendran-Nair and Tommy TY Lam

Abstract

The relationship among microbes, animals, and humans often manifests as zoonotic, anthropo-zoonotic, or sylvatic infections. Infections transmitted from animals to humans are considered zoonotic and often cause outbreaks of diseases, epidemics, or even pandemics. The battle for survival between microbes and mammalian species has been occurring throughout all documented human history. The control, de-escalation, or deceleration of the spread of these diseases often hinges upon the detection of infectious agents. The diagnostic tests to detect and monitor infectious agents have evolved throughout human biomedical history. Infectious disease diagnosis in the past decades has improved by combining physical examination, microbiology, immunology, and molecular tests. This chapter highlights the characteristics of diseases by their clinical presentation, laboratory tests, use of multi-omics, and other attributes of diagnostics.

Keywords: disease patterns, surveillance, diagnosis, laboratory technology, zoonosis

1. Introduction

Different surveillance systems have evolved throughout history to identify an array of traumatic zoonotic diseases that occur via cross-infection from animal to animal and animal to human. When a virus causes an animal disease, the same infectious agent can also be transmitted to humans. Thus, diagnostic tests in animals and humans are key to controlling the spread of diseases. An example is the availability of serological testing to diagnose vector-borne Eastern Equine Encephalitis Virus (EEEV). The virus is maintained in a cycle between birds and mosquitoes. The virus spreads among the species when mosquitoes feed on birds and mammals. The virus can cause long-term neurological damage and can be lethal to horses and humans—representing a public health threat to the region of the northeastern United

 IntechOpen

States. As a reportable disease, a positive test in horses prompts state surveillance to control infection. In addition, sentinel chickens and other poultries are serologically tested for the presence of the virus. Laboratory tests play a significant role in detecting and monitoring disease transmission.

The zoonotic diseases in this chapter illustrate the variety and evolution of laboratory and diagnostic tests. Diseases that are "zoonotic" are defined by the World Health Organization as "any diseases or infection that are naturally transmitted from vertebrate animals to humans." Researchers and authors have used zoonosis to describe infections or diseases transmitted from animals to humans. Additionally, sylvatic infection describes zoonotic infections from wild, non-domesticated animals to humans. This chapter highlights the discussion of each disease by its clinical signs in humans and animals, the origin of infection, the mode of transmission, and the laboratory diagnostic tests used.

1.1 Methodology and material

The clinical signs, infection origin, mode of transmission, and diagnostic tools have been determined for each disease based on scoping reviews of relevant literature published through PubMed. The review search with PubMed used the criteria: articles published in the past 10 years, the keywords "history," "diagnosis," and the specific disease names. Authors' experiences in clinical settings, microbiology, and research laboratories have also been included. This chapter is not a systematic review of all relevant publications. The intention of this chapter is to provide an overview of selected zoonotic agents that reside in food-producing animals, companion animals, and wildlife, as well as relevant diagnostic tests in the past decade.

2. Bacteroides

2.1 Anthrax

2.1.1 Human infections

Bacillus anthracis causes anthrax in humans and animals. It is a spore-forming, gram-positive bacterium. There was an outbreak in 2001 as a result of terrorism and multiple natural outbreaks including one in Texas in 2017 in the United States of America [1].

Human anthrax has been classified as agriculture or industrial anthrax.

The disease can be endemic in livestock and the environment. *Bacillus* can cause an acute infection that affects grazing livestock, wild ungulates, and human health [2]. The infection can manifest in three forms, involving the respiratory, gastroenteric, and cutaneous systems [3, 4].

The microbe can also exist in spores in meat or other foods that have been insufficiently cooked or in materials that have come into contact with contaminated animal products, such as wool or hair, which have undergone improper industrial processing [5]. The incubation period for anthrax is about 2–5 days according to World Health Organization, and 1–17 days per study by Doganay et al. The cutaneous form of anthrax is characterized by fever, hemorrhagic bullous lesions surrounded by extensive erythema, edema, leukocytosis, and possible toxemic shock. The gastroenteric form can cause acute septic shock and mortality [3].

2.1.2 Animal infections

Occurrences of the disease anthrax have been documented since 700 BC [6]. The first clinical documentation was described in 1752. The disease in animals can be acute, subacute, and chronic. The apoplectic form of anthrax is seen in cattle, sheep, and goats. The apoplectic form occurs most frequently at the beginning of an outbreak. Anthrax in animals occurs suddenly and leads to rapid death.

The symptoms of anthrax in animals consist of fever, recumbency, trembling, and dyspnea [6]. Blood fails to clot, and bloody discharges occur from orifices [6]. Chronic anthrax occurs in less susceptible species such as pigs. It has also been seen in cattle, horses, and dogs. During an outbreak in the herd of swine, some pigs will fall victim to the acute form, but most will suffer from chronic anthrax. The main symptom of the chronic form is pharyngeal and lingual edema. Foamy discharge from the mouth can be observed, and these animals can die from asphyxiation. Intestinal anthrax can also occur in pigs, presenting as localized chronic lesions. Anthrax can cause mortality in all previously mentioned animals and free-roaming wild animals.

2.1.3 Sources of infection and mode of transmission

The sources of human anthrax infection include infected animals, contaminated animal products, or environmental contamination. Cutaneous anthrax can be contracted from the process of skinning or butchering animals [5]. It can also be contracted by coming into contact with infected animal products. Pulmonary anthrax can be contracted from inhaling spores from a contaminated carcass or an animal hair [7]. These transmission modes have been observed in Asia, Africa, Australia, and North and South America [8]. Usually, in these cases, animals contract the infection by ingesting grass or water contaminated with spores. An animal dying from anthrax will produce large amounts of *B. anthrax* in their tissue. If their carcass is opened, the spores will contaminate the environment, including soil, grass, and water [9].

2.1.4 Diagnostic tests

Anthrax is considered a re-emerging disease. Anthrax in animals is diagnosed by laboratory tests that look for anthrax bacteria or antibodies in the animal's blood or other tissues. A review of susceptibility testing described that most anthrax strains are susceptible to first-line antimicrobials, though there are strains resistant to first-line antimicrobials [10].

Anthrax can also be suspected when an animal dies suddenly without prior symptoms, especially in ruminants. Other signs of anthrax include a rapidly decomposing carcass, bloody discharges from the nose, mouth, or anus, lack of rigor mortis, dark, tarlike un-clotted blood, or an enlarged spleen with a "blackberry jam" consistency. When collecting samples, care must be taken to avoid contaminating the environment and exposing people to the bacteria.

Historically, diagnosis can be confirmed by microscopic examination of stained smears of blood, pleural or ascites fluid, or lesion exudate depending on the route of infection, edema fluid in swine, and blood in other animals [6]. The *bacilli* can be cultured from liquid aspired from pustules or the blood of animals. The fluorescent antibody technique can be applied to fresh stains or blood smears. In another study, serum samples were used to detect IgG titers of the *bacilli* using enzyme-linked immunosorbent assay [11].

2.2 Botulism

2.2.1 Human infections

Botulism is considered a rare but life-threatening disease in humans [12]. Botulism poisoning occurs with ingestion of toxins produced by *Clostridium botulinum*. There are cases recorded in Europe as early as between 1967 and 1970. In Argentina, between 1967 and 1981, 139 cases were reported. In Poland, mortality occurred in 1.5 cases per 100,000 inhabitants between 1958 and 1969 [13]. Infant Botulism has been identified in the United States, Canada, Europe, and Australia. The first case of wound Botulism, occurring when a wound is contaminated by *Clostridium botulinum*, was recognized in 1943 by the Centers for Disease Control in the United States of America. Wound botulism can be presented with some clinical signs that are similar to classic Botulism [14].

Botulism is a neurotoxin, which can cause fatal respiratory failure. Therefore, during treatment, intubation and mechanical ventilation are often needed in conjunction with botulism antitoxin administration [12]. Botulism can also present as gastrointestinal symptoms, such as nausea, vomiting, and abdominal pain [15]. Patients can also exhibit neurological signs including diplopia and dysarthria [16, 17].

2.2.2 Animal infection

Botulism is economically important, particularly in livestock. Botulism cases have been recorded genomically in South Africa and Australia [18]. Botulism can occur in sheep, horses, and cattle and has been diagnosed in Europe, the United States of America, Australia, and South Africa. Botulism in horses can be both enteric and neurotoxic [19]. Botulism has been recorded in wild birds [20].

The main symptom of botulism in animals is partial or complete paralysis of the locomotor and swallowing muscles. The animals are described to be in a stupor or are obtunded for prolonged periods [21]. As the disease progresses, the animals cannot hold up their heads and experience recumbency, dysphagia, respiratory distress, and death. Sheep and cows typically present with the described symptoms. Horse's clinical signs also include muscle weakness, recumbency, decreased tail and tongue tone, respiratory distress, and death [22].

2.2.3 Source of infection and route of transmission

C. botulinum can be found in soil, dust, water, sediments, and vegetation. It can also be found in the intestine and liver of infected ducks [23]. Botulism outbreaks have also been reported on cattle farms infected by poultry [24]. It has been reported that contaminated feed, animal feces, and intestines of the infected animals are carriers of the disease [25]. After ingestion of *C. botulinum*, the toxin is absorbed through the intestines and circulated to the nervous system. Conversely, wound botulism is a result of environmental contamination [20].

2.2.4 Diagnosis

The most sensitive and widely accepted assay method for botulinum toxin is mouse bioassay, which takes 4 days to complete. As no rapid laboratory tests are available for botulism diagnosis, the therapy and notification of public health authorities must be based on clinical suspicions. Public health authorities must be notified of any suspected cases. Mouse bioassays, cell-based assays, immune assays, nucleic acid testing endopeptidase mass spectrometry assays, genomic comparative methods, and electrochemical detection and biosensors are assays with different time requirements and sensitivity [26].

A host of laboratory tests for botulism include microbiology, immunology, and molecular tests [27]. The virulence factor for botulism is a protein toxin, thus precluding other sensitive laboratory tests, such as polymerase chain reaction (PCR) amplification, usually employed for bacterial and viral pathogens. Three assays are highlighted by citation matching: enzyme-linked immunosorbent assay (ELISA), high-throughput fluorogenic assay, botulinum PCR-based assay, and most recently, fluorescent-based assay for botulinum neurotoxin protease activity [28].

Botulism is diagnosed in animals by clinical signs, laboratory tests, process of elimination, reproducibility of symptoms in animal models, and electrophysiological tests. Clinical signs require a veterinarian to examine the animal and take a history of exposure to risk factors. Symptoms of botulism include progressive muscle weakness, paralysis, and difficulty eating or drinking. Laboratory tests include blood, stool, and vomit samples that can be tested for the botulinum toxin. ELISA testing can be used to test large numbers of samples. Eliminating other causes of motor paralysis must be ruled out.

2.3 Brucellosis

2.3.1 Human infections

The main species in the genus of Brucellosis that infect humans are *Brucellosis abortus* and *Brucellosis suis*. These infections usually affect humans who have contact with goats and sheep through their occupations.

The incubation period can be anywhere from 1 week to many months. The disease can cause the sudden onset of localized abdominal pain and is accompanied by continued, intermittent, or regular pyrexia [29]. Brucellosis can present itself as pyrexia and fatigue, and can also cause anorexia, headache, irritation, depression, lymphadenopathy, splenomegaly, and hepatomegaly. Serious encephalitis, meningitis, neuritis, arthritis, and endocarditis can occur [29].

2.3.2 Animal infections

Bovine brucellosis has been eradicated in most European countries, Canada, the United States, Australia, and New Zealand [30]. Swine brucellosis is enzootic in Latin America. Goat and sheep brucellosis is a significant problem in Europe, Africa, and the Middle East. Ram epididymitis caused by *Brucellosis ovis* has been documented in New Zealand, Australia, Africa, Europe, and the United States. Infection of dogs with *Brucellosis canis* has been identified ubiquitously in various countries [31].

Natural brucellosis infections are difficult to diagnose. The symptoms in pregnant female cattle include spontaneous abortion, premature birth, stillbirth, or weak calves. Abortion usually occurs during the second half of pregnancy. Male and female calves less than 6 months of age are not susceptible to transitory infections. Thurs, calves infected through breast milk or contaminated food can eliminate brucellosis infections [32]. Brucellosis leading to retained placenta and metritis has been documented in laboratory animals and wildlife [33, 34]. Infection in swine can cause spontaneous abortions, infertility, the birth of weak piglets, orchitis, epididymitis, and arthritis. Infected piglets can retain infection and become carriers. Goats infected with *Brucella* spp. will also suffer from spontaneous abortion, in addition to symptoms of mastitis, which differs from other infected animals. In sheep, classic brucellosis and ram epididymitis are common [35].

2.3.3 Source of infection and route of transmission

Humans are infected by animals through direct contact with an infected animal, or indirectly by ingestion of infected animal products, or inhalation of airborne agents. Oral ingestion of raw cheese or milk from goats and sheep infected with *B. melitensis* is the most common origin of human brucellosis infection. Brucellae are resistant to the pickling or curing processes; therefore, ingesting game meat infected with *B. suis* can lead to human infection. Occupational infection in workers can be due to contact with infected animals in slaughterhouses, farms, or veterinary clinical settings.

Vaginal discharge, afterbirth, and fetuses are the main sources of infection among cattle. Cows that lick afterbirth, fetuses, newborn calves, or contaminated areas can ingest *Brucella* bacteria [36]. Infected males can transmit brucellosis to females. The same route of transmission occurs in swine, goats, sheep, and dogs.

2.3.4 Diagnosis

Yagupsky et al. describe laboratory diagnosis of human brucellosis. The tests include microbiological culture, serological tests, and nucleic acid amplification assays [37]. Cases with repeated exposure are difficult to diagnose based on serological tests [37].

Two types of tests can be conducted on animals. The first test category is "direct tests," which can be conducted on samples from animals with clinical signs. Indirect tests are for subclinical or suspected cases. Samples can be taken from lymph nodes, cerebrospinal fluid (CSF), and abscesses. Direct tests can be conducted by bacterial isolation, identification, and molecular methods. This includes conventional and real-time PCR, multiple-locus variable-number tandem repeat analysis, multi-locus sequence typing, and luminex multi-analyte profiling technology [38]. Indirect tests include milk ring test, buffered Brucella serological antigen test, rose Bengal test, buffered plate agglutination test, serum agglutination test, complement fixation test, indirect and competitive enzyme-linked immunosorbent assays [39], fluorescence polarization assay, immunoprecipitation tests, and lateral flow immunochromatography [38].

2.4 Clostridium

2.4.1 Human infections

Clostridium difficile is ubiquitous in the environment, animals, and human [40]. The environment, animals, including farm animals, companion animals, and food, are sources of human infection [41]. *Clostridium perfringens*, *novyi*, *septicum*, and *fallax* can infect wounds and lead to gas gangrene. Gas gangrene has been documented in both humans and animals [42]. A study in 2020 reported clostridium myonecrosis as a very rare but life-threatening necrotizing soft tissue infection [43]. Weese suggested that *Clostridium difficile* is a zoonotic pathogen due to the intra- and inter-species strain differences in humans and animals, but there is limited direct evidence of animal-human transmission [44]. Kachrimanidou et al. described shared ribotypes between animals and humans, therefore alluding to the zoonotic potential of *C. difficile* infection [45].

2.4.2 Animal infections

Clostridium perfringens Type A is a pathogenic strain that produces alpha toxin. In goats, *Clostridium septicum* has been reported to lead to sudden death [46]. In horses, *C. sordellii* has been reported to cause myonecrosis, cellulitis, and systemic changes suggestive of toxic shock [47]. Additionally, lambs with clostridium can suffer from depression, anemia, jaundice, and hemoglobinuria. *C. perfringens* Type A can cause death in lambs [48]. Type B can cause neonatal lamb death with abdominal bloating and hemorrhagic diarrhea [49]. *C. perfringens* Type C causes enterotoxemia in adult sheep and hemorrhagic enteritis in calves, lambs, and piglets. *C. perfringens* Type D causes enterotoxemia in sheep. *C. perfringens* Type E causes dysentery or enterotoxemia in calves and lambs [50].

2.4.3 Source of infection and route of transmission

The natural reservoir of *C. perfringens* type A is from environmental soil and the intestines of humans and animals. Clostridia that leads to wound infection is normally found in soil and intestinal tracts of animals. Transmission is facilitated by open wounds. Another route of infection for humans and animals is the oral-fecal route [51].

2.4.4 Diagnosis

Laboratory confirmation can be concluded by identifying the quantity of *C. perfringens* in food or fecal samples [52]. Serotyping in food and feces can assist with diagnosis. Other methods of diagnosis include detection of enterotoxin in patients' feces. Since the 1990s, Clostridium toxins can be diagnosed by agglutination, counter immunoelectrophoresis, and enzyme-linked immunosorbent assay (ELISA) [53].

2.5 Erysipelas

2.5.1 Human infections

Erysipeloid rhusiopathiae (E. rhusiopathiae) is a facultative anaerobe gram-positive bacteria. In humans, *E. rhusiopathiae* can cause bacteremia in immunocompromised patients [54]. It is an occupational disease occurring in slaughterhouses, poultry plants, and fish processing plants. *Erysipelas* infection can lead to erythematous, an edematous skin lesion with violet coloration around the lesion. Intense pruritus and pain can occur at the lesion site. The course of disease is usually not serious and patients recover in 2–4 weeks. However, if an infection becomes systemic, septicemia and endocarditis may cause death [55]. Tarasov et al. identified an antibiotic-resistant gene that highlighted the concern of not only the zoonotic nature of Erysipelothrix but also the risk of cross-species livestock and human infection [56].

2.5.2 Swine infections

Swine erysipelas is an economically important disease in exporting countries. Different strains of *Erysipelothrix* species have been isolated depending on the geographic location of the swine, the source of samples, and the diagnostic power of tests. McNeil et al. identified serotypes 1a, 1b, and 2 [57]. Pigs infected with *E. rhusiopathiae* Met-203 strains in Japan display arthritis, endocarditis, and urticaria [58].

2.5.3 Source of infection and mode of transmission

The principal reservoir for infection is swine, with fish and crustaceans as additional important sources of infection. Human erysipeloid occurs through the handling of these species with wound and skin abrasions.

2.5.4 Diagnosis

Erysipelas diagnosis relies on clinical signs, lesion observation, microscopy, polymerase chain reaction assay, and immunochemical and serological tests [59]. Complement fixation can be more useful in the diagnosis of cases with low titers, subclinical infection, and vaccination [59].

2.6 Leptospirosis

2.6.1 Human infections

Leptospirosis interrogans (L. interrogans) is a spirochete microbe that exists in over 180 serological variants or serovars [60]. Epidemic outbreaks are often caused by exposure to water contaminated with the urine of infected animals or exposure of an open wound to infected urine. The incubation period can last between 1 and 2 weeks. There are two types of infections. The first is the hepato-nephritic or icteric form, where jaundice and flu-like symptoms can occur. The second type is the anicteric form, which causes hemorrhagic urine and acute renal failure [61]. The icteric form presents with sudden onset of pyrexia, headache, lymphadenopathy, conjunctivitis, skin rash, nausea, vomiting, and diarrhea [62]. Hepatomegaly and jaundice are estimated to occur in 92% of the cases. Leptospirosis can lead to acute kidney injury with azotemia and nephrotic syndrome [63].

2.6.2 Animal infections

Leptospirosis pomona, *hardjo*, and *Grippotyphosa* are the common serovar in cattle. The clinical signs are not apparent in cattle [64]. The infection can cause pyrexia for a few days, anorexia, conjunctivitis, diarrhea, and a sudden decrease in milk production [65]. Cattle of all ages are susceptible. In a case study of a farm with mixed species livestock, 33% of swine and 12% of cattle population were infected [66]. *Leptospirosis pomona*, *Grippotyphosa*, *canicola*, and *icterohaemorrhagiae* are commonly identified in pigs and can lead to abortion and stunted piglet growth [67]. Infected equine species can also suffer from hepatonephritic, cardiovascular, ophthalmia, and reproductive symptoms [68].

Sheep and goats can also be infected by *L. Grippotyphosa* and *pomona, which can lead to pyrexia, anorexia, jaundice, hemoglobinuria, anemia, infertility, abortion*, the birth of weak offspring, or stillborn animals [69]. Dogs can be infected and remain asymptomatic. Dogs also can experience severe morbidity, with 10% mortality. They may develop a sudden onset of pyrexia, hemorrhages, necrosis, and pharyngitis. Icterus may develop with infection by the *L. icterohaemorrhagiae* serovar. Cases in cats have been rarely reported. Rodents are a natural host of *Leptospirosis*, therefore, they are asymptomatic even when infected. *Leptospira* can infect a wide range of mammalian species. Golden Syrian hamsters, guinea pigs, and gerbils are sensitive to acute disease and can be used as animal models [69, 70]. Adult rabbits are resistant to *Leptospirosis* infection and are a species of choice for antibody production [69].

2.6.3 Source of infection and route of transmission

Animals such as rats can harbor *Leptospirosis* spp. and shed leptospires in their urine. The urine contaminates the environment and directly or indirectly infects human and animals by skin, oral, nasal, and conjunctival mucosa. Indirect exposure through water, soil, or foods contaminated by infected animals is a common route of transmission.

2.6.4 Diagnosis

Bacteria can be isolated from the bodily fluids or feces of infected individuals by polymerase chain reaction (PCR) [69]. It has been diagnosed from sites of the kidney, lung, and pleural fluid of anicteric fetuses [64].

There are high levels of diversity in the leptospiral strain. A study applied PCR of lipL32 gene to identify leptospiral DNA in the thymus, lungs, heart, subcapsular kidney, liver, kidneys, and abomasal liquid. Only one fetus' kidney and liver contained leptospiral DNA [71].

Testing can be done with the direct culture of urine, or the direct culture of blood 1 week after infection of the infected animal. Hamster model inoculations have been described in multiple publications [72]. In the leptospiremia stage and the acute stage, leptospires can be recovered in blood or bodily fluids. Following the leptospiremia stage is the leptospirosis stage when leptospires are excreted in urine with an IgM antibody increase [73].

2.7 Lyme disease

2.7.1 Human infections

"Lyme arthritis" is caused by spirochete *Borrelia burgdorferi*. It was identified in 1977 in Lyme, Connecticut, United States of America. It has been identified in the United States, Europe, and Australia [74]. The distribution of disease is associated with the presence of the vector, tick of the *Ixodes ricinus* complex. Between 1975 and 1979, 242 cases were documented in Lyme, CT. There have been about 476,000 cases identified in the United States, and upward of 200,000 cases in Western Europe [75].

The disease is described as multistage, multisystem, acute, chronic, and noncontagious inflammatory [69]. The characteristic cutaneous lesion such as erythema chronicum migrants appears between 3 and 20 days after the tick bite. The lesion is characterized by clearly delineated borders, with a pale center and annular erythema. The clinical signs can include carditis, keratitis, uveitis, and arthritis [76].

2.7.2 Animal infections

Between 1978 and 1982, tick *Ixodes dammini* was identified in the state of Connecticut in the United States in white-footed mice, chipmunks, squirrels, opossums, raccoons, and dogs. Animals are considered responsible for maintaining the infection in natural foci.

2.7.3 Source of infection and route of transmission

Transmission is by *Ixodes* ticks although alternative agents were considered [69]. The larvae tick is not infected with Lyme disease when they hatch. They become infected when they feed on infected animals. Transmission occurs mostly between animals and ticks, with humans as incidental hosts.

2.7.4 Diagnosis

Diagnosis in the 1980s was conducted by culture. Serology tests, including enzyme-linked immunosorbent assays (ELISA), indirect immunofluorescence tests with conjugated IgM and IgG sera, and Western immunoblots, are used in diagnosis [69, 77].

2.8 Tuberculosis

2.8.1 Human infections

Tuberculosis is caused by *Mycobacterium tuberculosis* complex species. Cattle is the primary host of *Mycobacterium bovis*, which poses a zoonotic risk. The prevalence of human tuberculosis of animal origin has been reduced, especially in countries where mandatory pasteurization of milk has been implemented.

M. bovis can cause the same clinical forms and pathologic lesions as *Mycobacterium tuberculosis*. Historically, the most prevalent forms caused by *M. bovis* were extra-pulmonary. Extrapulmonary tuberculosis can appear as pericarditis, genital urinary infections, tuberculosis of bones and joints, and meningitis [78]. Pulmonary tuberculosis caused by bovine bacillus occurs less frequently, but significantly in occupational groups in contact with infected cattle or their carcasses [79].

Humans who suffer from pulmonary tuberculosis of bovine origin can re-transmit the infection to cattle. The most recent publication of human-to-cattle *Mycobacterium tuberculosis* complex transmission occurred in the United States [80]. Cattle are resistant to *M. tuberculosis* but the bacillus can survive in the bovine tissue and lymph nodes. Thus, the cattle can be interpreted as positive on diagnostic tests.

2.8.2 Animal infections

In industrialized countries, bovine tuberculosis has been eradicated, or is in the advanced stage of control. However, the situation has not improved in some regions, such as in locations where milk products remain unpasteurized, which can increase disease incidence. The infection rate in swine is similar to or even higher than in cattle if there is cross-contamination from swine feed. One study indicates cattle-to-cattle transmission of bovine tuberculosis [81].

The main agent for cattle tuberculosis is *M. bovis*. Calves can be infected by contaminated milk. However, inhalation is the most common clinical and pathological form. The bacillus enters the lungs, multiplies, and forms a primary focus. From the foci, the bacillus can enter the lymph node on the infected lung's ipsilateral side, forming a primary complex [81]. When the animal's immune system can no longer keep the bacillus in the primary foci, the bacillus travels to other organs through the lymphatic and vascular system, which causes generalized infection. Some of the infections remain subclinical, and the animal remains asymptomatic. Other animals develop bronchopneumonia, which is presented with coughing, weight loss, and reduced milk production. Dyspnea can occur when lung tissues are compromised by the bacillus. Cattle are very resistant to *M. tuberculosis* and normally do not produce anatomically identifiable lesions.

Swine are susceptible to *M. bovis*, *M. avium-intracellulare*, and *M. tuberculosis*. *M. bovis* is the most pathogenic and invasive for swine. Gastrointestinal infection can be caused by the consumption of milk or milk products. The primary infection complex is found in the oropharynx and the submaxillary lymph nodes, or the intestine and the mesenteric lymph node. It is found that *M. bovis* causes more severe clinical symptoms compared to *M. tuberculosis*. The clinical signs of *M. bovis* include dyspnea, inappetence, and acute death, compared to swine experimentally infected with *M. tuberculosis* that remained bright, alert, and with good appetite [82].

Sheep and goats were found to be infected mainly with *M. avium* in 1970 [83]. Sheep that shared pasture with cattle were infected with *M. bovis*, bovine tuberculosis [84]. Conversely, horses rarely contract tuberculosis. Companion animals such as felines and canines are resistant to experimental tuberculosis [85]. Captive animals in zoos, farms, laboratories, and homes can be exposed to infection [86].

The history of captive non-human primates in TB research is described by Scanga et al. Scanga models that TB is not biphasic but a continuum of caseous, fibrocalcific, sclerotic, or mineralized lesions and symptoms [87]. Humans can transmit the bacillus to several animal species, mainly non-human primates and canines, producing progressive tuberculosis. The maintenance host in wildlife can include goats, buffalo, deer, bison, elk, moose, badgers, and possums [88].

2.8.3 Source of infection and mode of transmission

The principal reservoir of *M. bovis* is cattle. Cattle can transmit the infection to many mammals, including humans. Humans can contract the disease by ingesting raw milk and milk products or inhaling the bacillus. Tuberculosis is transmitted between cattle via aerosol [89]. Additionally, vertical transmission in animals by the digestive route can occur before weaning. Sylvatic transmission from wildlife to domestic animals, and subsequently domestic animals to wildlife has been recorded. Cattle, fowl, and sometimes humans are the principal transmission routes for swine, goats, and sheep [90].

2.8.4 Diagnosis

A systematic review by Taye et al. described genotyping-based studies that reported a significantly lower prevalence of zoonotic TB than those using older techniques [91].

The gold standard of diagnosis is the culture of the agent. The routine diagnosis of tuberculosis in cattle is through the tuberculin skin test (TST). Studies compare conventional PCR, real-time PCR, isothermal DNA amplification, and nanotechnologies. The recommendation for speed of diagnosis is to combine classical and molecular diagnostics to facilitate disease tracking [92].

Mantoux test can be used to diagnose tuberculosis by intracutaneous or intradermal injection. The QuantiFERON test of the interferon-gamma in the plasma (International Unit per milliliter) tests for *M. tuberculosis* with a higher sensitivity and specificity [93]. The spontaneous outbreak of *Mycobacterium tuberculosis* complex infection among captive primates in research facilities prompted a study of testing algorithms. The author suggested four parameters to improve the testing of TB cases. The algorithm includes clinical assessment, antibody titer to assess humoral immunity, TST and interferon-gamma assay to assess cell-mediated immunity, and agent detection by PCR at necropsy of captive primates from high-TB-risk regions [94].

3. Viral

3.1 Herpesvirus simiae infection

3.1.1 Human infections

The B virus, Cercopithecine herpesvirus 1 or Macacine Herpesvirus 1, is a macaque alpha-herpes virus that is antigenically related to herpes simplex virus and SA-8 (a baboon and *Cercopithecus* sp. herpesvirus). It is a DNA virus of the subfamily Alphaherpesvirinae in the family of Herpesviridae.

The disease occurs in humans who handle non-human primates or their tissues in research centers or in vaccine production plants. The first documented case of human B virus infection was documented in 1932 when a researcher was bitten on the hand by a clinically asymptomatic rhesus macaque (*Macaca mulatta*) and died of progressive encephalomyelitis [95].

Herpesvirus simiae produces a highly fatal disease in humans. Historically, the incubation period was thought to be 1–5 weeks. However, recent cases describe a shorter incubation period (https://www.cdc.gov/herpes-b-virus/about/index.html). The bite or scratch from a non-human primate infected with herpesvirus simiae can lead to vesiculation at the wound site, followed by lymphadenitis. The patient will experience pyrexia, cephalgia, nausea, abdominal pain, and diarrhea. Encephalitis or encephalomyelitis can last between 3 and 21 days [96].

3.1.2 Animal infections

Reviews of the herpes simplex virus-like alpha-herpesvirus of non-human primates indicate that B virus of natural host in macaque can cross-infect humans. HVP2 in baboons can cause fatal cross-infection in colobus monkeys, and HVS1 in squirrel monkeys can cross-infect and cause fatal disease in owl monkeys, marmosets, and humans [97].

The infection in non-human primates produces a benign disease that can be subclinical or clinical. The disease appears similar to that produced by herpes hominins in humans. The most common lesions are localized in the mouth on the tongue. The ulcerations can be covered with a fibrinous necrotic scab, and the symptoms can last between 7 and 14 days. The lesions do not leave scars or affect the condition of the animal [69]. The herpetiform eruption can occur on the mucocutaneous border of the lips and sometimes on the conjunctiva and skin. The lesions may not be noticeable per cage-side observation.

3.1.3 Source of infection and mode of transmission

The main source of infection is rhesus monkey (*Macaca mulatta*). Other monkeys of the same genus can be a source of human infection. The modes of transmission include bites or skin abrasions contaminated with monkey saliva, or infected aerosol that enters through the conjunctiva, nose, or pharynx. Injuries related to working with macaques can mean exposure to Simiae Alpha-herpes virus [98].

3.1.4 Diagnosis

The ELISA methodologies provide a rapid diagnostic tool with increased detection, sensitivities, and enhanced specificity when competition protocols are utilized. The antibodies that develop in response to herpes B virus infection in both humans and non-human primates can neutralize HSV-1 and HSV-2 and non-human primate alpha herpesviruses [99]. Differentiation of herpes simplex, herpes hominins, and SA-8 is difficult because of antigenic similarities [97].

3.2 Influenza

3.2.1 Human infections

The influenza virus is an RNA genome virus from the family of Orthomyxoviridae.

Influenza occurs in epidemic form and is characterized by high morbidity and low mortality. Large epidemics and pandemics occurred in 1918, 1957, 1968, and 2000. These epidemics and pandemics were largely due to Type A influenza. Type B influenza generally causes less extensive epidemics than Type A [100].

Respiratory symptoms such as nasal obstruction, coughing, and sneezing can be present at the onset of the viral illness. Diarrhea and abdominal pain are reported but uncommon. High-grade fevers have been associated with influenza. Respiratory signs and symptoms usually become more intense as pyrexia increases. The duration of pyrexia ranges from 3 to 5 days [101].

3.2.2 Animal infections

Swine influenza has been known since 1918 when it first appeared and was documented in the Midwest United States. Within a period of 3–4 months of that year, millions of swine became ill and subsequently died [102]. In 1979, H1N1 was identified in an episodic swine influenza outbreak in Belgium [103]. In horses, equine influenza can be caused by subtypes of type A (H7N7) [104]. The second subtype in horses (H3N8) was isolated in the United States, Canada, Uruguay, and Brazil [104]. In birds, numerous subtypes of the virus have been found, which suggest the potential for antigenic recombination with evidence of antigenic drift [101]. During the winter of 1978 to 1980 on the Cape Cod peninsula, United States of America, harbor seals (*Phoca vitulina*) were found deceased with H7N7 isolates from lungs with high titers, and brains with low titers [105]. Felines can be experimentally infected with human H3N2 that caused the pandemic in 1968 [106]. H3N2 was isolated from canines in Taiwan [107]. H3N2 and H1N1 have been isolated in canines in Italy and several other countries [108].

The symptoms in animals are similar to human symptoms. In swine, the disease is characterized by sudden onset of pyrexia, loss of appetite, coughing, nasal and ocular discharge, and dyspnea [109]. In birds, the infection can range from asymptomatic to death. In a study that inoculated young birds with the virus, the clinical signs were very mild, with the exception of one bird. The clinical signs in adult layers were more severe than in young chickens. A post-mortem study indicated splenomegaly, fibrinous to caseous exudate in the coelomic cavity in adult birds that were clinically healthy. Common signs of influenza in chickens are ruffled feathering and severe depression [110].

3.2.3 Source of infection and route of transmission

The Influenza virus can be transmitted by fomites, aerosols, or secretions from infected humans or animals [111].

3.2.4 Diagnosis

There are several approaches available for the diagnosis of influenza infections in humans. In the past two decades, molecular methods have been the mainstay in diagnosing influenza virus [109]. Diagnosis also includes viral isolation in cell culture, immunofluorescence assays, nucleic acid amplification tests, immunochromatography-based rapid diagnostic tests, immunohistochemistry (IHC), and RT-PCR. RT-PCR is effective for the initial diagnosis and has better sensitivity than other rapid assays. Whole genome sequencing can be performed, molecular assays can be used to subtype influenza isolates, and sequence analysis of hemagglutinin is used in surveillance studies and vaccine strain selection [112].

3.3 Rabies

3.3.1 Human infections

The rabies virus is an RNA virus belonging to the genus *Lyssavirus* of family Rhabdoviridae. It contains an internal nucleoprotein and an external glycoprotein service antigen that induces neutralizing antibodies. Outside of the United States, rabies infections have been reported in humans in South Africa, Africa, China, Ethiopia, Bali, India, and Thailand [113].

The bite of a rabid animal leads to infection in humans with an incubation period of 30–90 days [114]. The disease begins with anxiety and mild pyrexia. The patient usually feels pain and irritation in the region of the wound. The following excitation phase includes extreme sensitivity to light and sound, dilatation of pupils, and an increase in salivation. Swallowing dysfunction is seen in most patients [69]. Many patients also experience spasmodic laryngeal pharyngeal contractions. There may also be spasms of the respiratory muscles and generalized convulsions. The excitation phase may persist until death or be replaced by a generalized paralysis. The disease lasts 2–6 days and almost invariably ends in death [115].

3.3.2 Animal infections

The incubation period can be variable in animals. Viruses isolated from animals without modifications in the laboratory can be prolonged depending on the capacity to invade the salivary glands. By contrast, strains adapted to laboratory animals have a short incubation period of 4–6 days and do not invade the salivary gland [116].

Rabies in bats is a problem independent of the infection cycles in other mammals [117]. Insectivorous, omnivorous, and piscivorous bats that are non-hematophagus in North and South America are confirmed to carry rabies [118].

DOI: http://dx.doi.org/10.5772/intechopen.1008157

In animals, there are two forms of rabies—furious rabies and paralytic rabies—determined by the corresponding neurological signs [119]. The incubation period lasts from 10 days to 2 or more months. In canines in the prodromal phase, they may exhibit a behavioral change, hide in dark corners, show unusual agitation, and pace restlessly [115]. Rabid canines can appear easily startled and anorexic. After 1–3 days, the canine can become aggressive and salivate profusely. In the terminal phase of the disease, generalized convulsions are typically observed and followed by muscular incoordination and paralysis of the trunk and extremities. The paralytic form is characterized by predominately paralytic symptoms. The excitation phase is very short or absent. Paralysis begins with muscle of the head and neck region and the animal will have difficulty swallowing. The disease progresses to paralytic rabies of the extremities, general paralysis, and death. The course of the paralytic form has been documented to last 1–11 days [120].

Felines exhibit similar signs to canines. Cattle usually contract rabies from the vampire bat and tend to have a long incubation period. The predominant symptoms in cattle are paralysis, and the disease is known as paralytic bovine rabies. Affected animals stray away from the herd with dilated pupils and raised hair. Abnormal hindlimb movement can be observed. Muscle tremors, restlessness, and hypersensitivity in the wound area can also be observed. As the disease progresses, muscular incoordination and tonic-clonic contractions of the muscle groups of the neck, trunk, and extremities occur. The animal will have difficulty swallowing and cease rumination. The animal subsequently dies. Other animals, such as equines, ovines, and goats, experience symptoms similar to those of bovine rabies. The excitation phase can vary in length and intensity but the paralytic symptoms almost always occur, causing difficulty in swallowing and coordination of extremities [115].

3.3.3 Origin of infection and route of transmission

Animal hosts that maintain rabies virus in nature are carnivores and bats. Herbivores and other non-biting animals, such as rodents and lagomorphs, do not play any role in the epidemiology of the disease.

3.3.4 Diagnosis

The preferred test is the direct immunofluorescence test. In 1984a, the WHO recommended that when the test is introduced in a laboratory, an inoculation should be made in mice for a year. It is also recommended that the inoculation of mice with cerebral material from the suspected animal be carried out if the immunofluorescence test is negative. The fluorescence test can use samples from corneal impressions, scrapings of the lingual mucosa, bulbar tissue of the hair follicles, and frozen skin secretions. A positive result confirms the diagnosis. However, a negative result cannot exclude infection. This test can commence early prophylactic treatment of the exposed person.

By the same token, microscopic examination of Negri bodies can be useful for diagnosis. Experienced personnel can obtain a correct diagnosis using May-Grünwald and Mann stains or other techniques to confirm rabies infection. However, a negative finding does not rule out the possibility of infection. In these cases, neurological and salivary glands should be examined.

Diagnosing rabies infections is crucial; therefore, studies continue to improve diagnostic sensitivity and specificity, increase the speed, and decrease the costs of molecular and serology tests. Rasolonjatovo et al. looked at the sensitivity and specificity of the molecular tests using reverse transcription followed by a hemi-nested polymerase chain reaction of dried brain tissue as a field diagnostic test in low-resource or low-access settings [121]. Torquato et al. compared a direct fluorescent antibody test or viral isolation in a mouse inoculation test with a reverse transcription-polymerase chain reaction using (RT-qPCR) an indirect rapid immunohistochemistry test on equine samples of the central nervous system [122]. Approaches such as biosensor and RT-qPCR are being studied in different laboratories [123, 124].

3.4 Orthopoxvirus infections

3.4.1 Human infections

Human monkeypox is caused by the monkeypox virus which is an orthopoxvirus. There is a recurrence of monkeypox in the human population [125] and it is an emerging zoonotic disease according to the World Health Organization [126, 127]. The signs and symptoms of monkeypox in humans bear resemblance to human smallpox. The human patient is usually pyrexic and has a rash and swollen lymph nodes [126]. It is usually a self-limiting disease with more severe symptoms and complications in children. The eruption of skin lesions is more frequent on the face and extremities than on the body trunk. The conjunctiva and cornea may also be affected [128].

An Orthopoxvirus causes smallpox. Smallpox was classified by the density of the rash in the 1870s. In 1958, the World Health Organization started a smallpox eradication program, and the disease has been eradicated with no natural cases since the 1970s.

3.4.2 Animal infections

The smallpox virus causes infection with a historical context and a contemporary profile. It was first recognized in 1958, where in Europe and the United States of America, about 10 outbreaks were reported in captive non-human primates in research centers or zoos. No personnel cases had been reported who were in contact with these animals [129].

In captive non-human primates, lesions have been observed to consist of multiple and discrete papules. Lesions are abundant on the palms of the hands, the trunk, and the tail. The common marmoset model identified the orthopoxvirus infection, and fatal infection has been reported in New World monkeys [130].

3.4.3 Source of infection and mode of transmission

Historically, smallpox spread rapidly. It made history by causing epidemics across Europe, Asia, and America [131]. There is a major source of uncertainty in models used for public health planning. The mode of transmission is by mucosal contacts between individuals and person-to-person airborne droplets.

The monkeypox virus was considered to have low efficiency in human-to-human transmission. However, in October 2022, more than 76,000 confirmed cases of human monkeypox, in 102 countries, attracted attention to the control of the epidemic [132].

Cowpox virus is transmitted to humans through an infected animal and is low in pathogenicity. Camelpox virus has been confirmed by laboratories in India and Sudan [132].

3.4.4 Diagnosis

Diagnosis of smallpox by clinical signs can bear resemblance to chickenpox. Viruses can be isolated from skin lesions, including scabs. The isolated strains are usually sent to a reference laboratory to identify the variola virus. Under electron microscopy, the brick shape of the variola virus distinguishes it from varicella-zoster virus. A polymerase chain reaction assay for orthopoxviral genes can be used to identify variola virus.

Antibodies for monkeypox and smallpox viruses can be differentiated by cross-adsorption with heterologous antigens. Specific antibodies are detected by the immunodiffusion and immunofluorescence techniques. In the 1970s, radioimmunoassay was a simple process after one adsorption with antigenic preparations. It allowed direct measurement of the relative concentration of residual antibodies for each virus [133]. Suitable samples are surface lesions and skin materials such as exudates, swabs, and crusts. A laboratory can perform nucleic acid amplification, such as polymerase chain reaction. Positive detection using MPXV PCR assay in suspected cases, along with clinical history and epidemiology consideration, can confirm MPXV infection. Genetic sequence data (GSD) can provide additional information on the origin of the cases [133].

3.5 West Nile virus (WNV)

3.5.1 Human infections

West Nile fever is caused by West Nile virus, an RNA virus in the genus of *Flavivirus*, Togaviridae. The virus circulates among birds and through arthropods that feed on infected mammalian species. The virus has been isolated, and from serum neutralization, it can be determined that infections are present in humans, mammals, birds, and arthropods in Africa, Asia, Europe, the Middle East, America, and Australia [134].

Infection symptoms in humans can range from uncomplicated pyrexia to fatal meningoencephalitis [135]. The onset of the disease is acute, with pyrexia, ocular pain, muscular pain, joint pain, and gastrointestinal signs. Less frequent symptoms include myocarditis, meningitis, and encephalitis. The disease can be seasonal and occur more frequently during the summer when mosquitoes are more abundant. Climate change has altered the extrinsic incubation condition and led to the West Nile Epizootic Emergence in Germany in 2019 [136].

3.5.2 Animal infections

Among domestic animals, horses appear to be the only species that present with clinical manifestations [137]. A West Nile fever outbreak occurred between 1962 and 1964 among horses in France. It caused fatal encephalitis outbreaks in equine from 1996 to 2000 in Europe and Russia [69].

3.5.3 Source of infection and mode of transmission

West Nile virus is a zoonosis transmitted from birds to humans and other mammals through mosquitoes of the genus *Culex*. Humans, horses, sheep, and cattle are accidental dead-end virus hosts. Birds are a reservoir since they have high titers and prolonged viremia to serve as a source of infection for the arthropod vector. The virus has been isolated in pigeons (*Columba livia*) in Iran [138], and turtledoves (*Stretopelia turtur*) in Israel [139]. Ornithophilic mosquitoes of the genus *Culex* are a mode of transmission; they feed on the blood of a bird with viremia, and then the mosquito transmits the infection by biting a susceptible host, either bird or mammal.

3.5.4 Diagnosis

Three commonly used diagnostic methods include nucleic acid detection, enzyme-linked immunoassay (ELISA), and plaque reduction neutralization test (PRNT) [140]. Per a comparative study conducted in 2020, the VIRCLIA IgM and IgG mono test can qualitatively detect WNV in serum and CSF specimens [141].

4. Conclusion

A variety of laboratory tests are used to identify zoonotic infections. These tests apply microscopy, microbiology, serology, immunology, and multi-omics technology. By reviewing clinical signs in humans and animals, transmission modes, and origins of infection of bacterial and viral zoonotic agents, we describe the spectrum of disease presentation and the laboratory tests in diagnosing infectious agents. This is particularly significant as faster, more sensitive, more specific, and less costly diagnostic tests are ideal yet unavailable—or, if available, may not be universally accessible. An adaptive, systematic, and efficient reporting surveillance system would help control, monitor, and prevent zoonotic disease transmission.

Conflict of interest

The authors declare no conflict of interest.

Author details

Olivia Sinn Kay Chan[1]*, Meera Surendran-Nair[2] and Tommy TY Lam[3]

1 Institute of Comparative Medicine, Columbia University Irving Medical Center, New York, NY, USA

2 Antech Diagnostics, California, USA

3 Li Ka Shing Faculty of Medicine, The University of Hong Kong, Hong Kong

*Address all correspondence to: soc3@cumc.columbia.edu

IntechOpen

© 2024 The Author(s). Licensee IntechOpen. This chapter is distributed under the terms of the Creative Commons Attribution License (http://creativecommons.org/licenses/by/4.0), which permits unrestricted use, distribution, and reproduction in any medium, provided the original work is properly cited.

References

[1] Dacso MM et al. Texas professionals are employing a one health approach to protect the United States against biosecurity threats. One Health. 2022;**15**:100431

[2] Carlson CJ et al. The global distribution of *Bacillus anthracis* and associated anthrax risk to humans, livestock and wildlife. Nature Microbiology. 2019;**4**(8):1337-1343

[3] Hashemi SA et al. A case of fatal gastrointestinal anthrax in north eastern Iran. Case Reports in Infectious Diseases. 2015;**2015**:875829

[4] Hendricks K et al. Clinical features of patients hospitalized for all routes of Anthrax, 1880-2018: A systematic review. Clinical Infectious Diseases. 2022;**75**(Suppl. 3):S341-s353

[5] Doganay M et al. Human anthrax: Update of the diagnosis and treatment. Diagnostics. 2023;**13**(6):1056

[6] Alam ME et al. Review of anthrax: A disease of farm animals. Journal of Advanced Veterinary and Animal Research. 2022;**9**(2):323

[7] Ngetich W. Review of anthrax: A disease of animals and humans. International Journal of Agriculture, Environment and Bioresearch. 2019;**4**:123-134

[8] Sushma B et al. An estimate of global anthrax prevalence in livestock: A meta-analysis. Veterinary World. 2021;**14**(5):1263

[9] Sidwa T et al. Control and prevention of anthrax, Texas, USA, 2019. Emerging Infectious Diseases. 2020;**26**(12):2815

[10] Maxson T et al. Systematic review of in vitro antimicrobial susceptibility testing for *Bacillus anthracis*, 1947-2019. Clinical Infectious Diseases. 2022;**75**(Suppl. 3):S373-s378

[11] Gulseren D et al. Evaluation of clinical and serological findings for diagnosis of cutaneous anthrax infection after an outbreak. Cutaneous and Ocular Toxicology. 2017;**36**(3):289-293

[12] Rao AK et al. Clinical guidelines for diagnosis and treatment of botulism, 2021. MMWR - Recommendations and Reports. 2021;**70**(2):1-30

[13] Hauschild AHW. Epidemiology of human foodborne botulism. In: *Clostridium botulinum*. CRC Press; 2018. pp. 69-104. eBook ISBN9781315139623. DOI: 10.1201/9781315139623

[14] Chatham-Stephens K et al. Clinical features of foodborne and wound botulism: A systematic review of the literature, 1932-2015. Clinical Infectious Diseases. 2018;**66**(suppl. 1):S11-S16

[15] Min M et al. An outbreak of botulinum types A, B, and E associated with vacuum-packaged salted fish and ham. The Journal of Emergency Medicine. 2021;**60**(6):760-763

[16] Kuratle M et al. A case of sole supportive care of severe neuroparalytic foodborne botulism due to homemade pesto. Medizinische Klinik, Intensivmedizin und Notfallmedizin. 2019;**114**(1):59-62

[17] Gul Dar N et al. The first reported foodborne botulism outbreak in Riyadh, Saudi Arabia: Lessons learned. Journal

of Epidemiology and Global Health. 2024;**14**(3):1071-1076

[18] Smith TJ et al. Genomic characterization of newly completed genomes of Botulinum neurotoxin-producing species from Argentina, Australia, and Africa. Genome Biology and Evolution. 2020;**12**(3):229-242

[19] Uzal FA et al. Clostridial diseases of horses: A review. Vaccine. 2022;**10**(2):318

[20] Gutiérrez-Arnal J, Marín C. The latent threat in wild birds: *Clostridium botulinum*. Veterinary Sciences. 2024;**11**(1):36

[21] Mayhew J, MacKay R. Large Animal Neurology. UK: John Wiley & Sons; 2022

[22] Stratford C, Mayhew I, Hudson N. Equine botulism: A clinical approach to diagnosis and management. Equine Veterinary Education. 2014;**26**(8):441-448

[23] Nguyen DH, Nguyen TT, Nguyen HT. Investigation of botulism in free-range duck farming in the Mekong Delta, Vietnam. Open Veterinary Journal. 2022;**12**(5):632-638

[24] Souillard R et al. Occurrence of *C. botulinum* in healthy cattle and their environment following poultry botulism outbreaks in mixed farms. Veterinary Microbiology. 2015;**180**(1-2):142-145

[25] Espelund M, Klaveness D. Botulism outbreaks in natural environments—An update. Frontiers in Microbiology. 2014;**5**:287

[26] Centurioni DA, Egan CT, Perry MJ. Current developments in diagnostic assays for laboratory confirmation and investigation of botulism. Journal of Clinical Microbiology. 2022;**60**(4):e00139-20

[27] Malik YS, Milton AAP, Ghatak S, Ghosh S. Clostridial Infections (Avian Botulism). In: Role of Birds in Transmitting Zoonotic Pathogens. Singapore: Springer; 2021. pp. 115-124. DOI: 10.1007/978-981-16-4554-9

[28] Kolesnikov AV et al. Ultrasensitive detection of protease activity of anthrax and botulinum toxins by a new PCR-based assay. Pathogens and Disease. 2016;**74**(1):ftv112

[29] Young EJ. Clinical manifestations of human brucellosis. In: Brucellosis. CRC Press; 2020. pp. 97-126. eBook ISBN9781003068518

[30] Yasmin B, Lone S. Brucellosis: An economically important infection. Journal of Medical Microbiology and Diagnosis. 2015;**4**(208):1000208. DOI: 10.4172/2161-0703.1000208

[31] Corbel MJ. Brucellosis: Epidemiology and prevalence worldwide. In: Brucellosis. CRC Press; 2020. pp. 25-40. eBook ISBN9781003068518

[32] Deresa B, Tulu D, Deressa FB. Epidemiological investigation of cattle abortion and its association with brucellosis in Jimma zone, Ethiopia. Veterinary Medicine: Research and Reports. 2020;**11**:87-98

[33] Wang Z et al. A pregnant mouse model for the vertical transmission of *Brucella melitensis*. The Veterinary Journal. 2014;**200**(1):116-121

[34] Ntirandekura J-B et al. Association of brucellosis with abortion prevalence in humans and animals in Africa: A review. African Journal of Reproductive Health. 2018;**22**(3):120-136

[35] Saxena N, Singh BB, Saxena HM. Brucellosis in sheep and goats and its serodiagnosis and epidemiology.

International Journal of Current Microbiology and Applied Sciences. 2018;7(1):1848-1877

[36] Kiros A, Asgedom H, Abdi RD. A review on bovine brucellosis: Epidemiology, diagnosis and control options. ARC Journal of Animal and Veterinary Sciences (AJAVS). 2016;**2**(3):8-21

[37] Yagupsky P, Morata P, Colmenero JD. Laboratory diagnosis of human brucellosis. Clinical Microbiology Reviews. 2019;**33**(1):10-1128. DOI: 10.1128/cmr.00073-19

[38] Saavedra MJ, Fernandes C, Queiroga C. Laboratory diagnosis of brucellosis. In: Brucellosis in Goats and Sheep: An Endemic and Re-emerging Old Zoonosis in the 21st Century. NY Nova Science Publisher; 2019. pp. 151-180. ISBN: 978-1-53614-962-3

[39] Praud A et al. Evaluation of three competitive ELISAs and a fluorescence polarisation assay for the diagnosis of bovine brucellosis. The Veterinary Journal. 2016;**216**:38-44

[40] Rodriguez Diaz C, Seyboldt C, Rupnik M. Non-human *C. difficile* reservoirs and sources: Animals, food, environment. Advances in Experimental Medicine and Biology. 2018;**1050**:227-243

[41] Di Bella S et al. *Clostridioides difficile* infection: History, epidemiology, risk factors, prevention, clinical manifestations, treatment, and future options. Clinical Microbiology Reviews. 2024;**37**(2):e0013523

[42] Liu S et al. Amentoflavone attenuates *Clostridium perfringens* gas gangrene by targeting alpha-toxin and perfringolysin O. Frontiers in Pharmacology. 2020;**11**:179

[43] Leiblein M et al. Clostridial gas gangrene—A rare but deadly infection: Case series and comparison to other necrotizing soft tissue infections. Orthopaedic Surgery. 2020;**12**(6):1733-1747

[44] Weese JS. Clostridium (Clostridioides) difficile in animals. Journal of Veterinary Diagnostic Investigation. 2020;**32**(2):213-221

[45] Kachrimanidou M, Tzika E, Filioussis G. Clostridioides (Clostridium) difficile in food-producing animals, horses and household pets: A comprehensive review. Microorganisms. 2019;**7**(12):667. DOI: 10.3390/microorganisms7120667

[46] Gazioglu A et al. Sudden death due to gas gangrene caused by *Clostridium septicum* in goats. BMC Veterinary Research. 2018;**14**:1-6

[47] Sacco SC et al. *Clostridium sordellii*–associated gas gangrene in 8 horses, 1998-2019. Journal of Veterinary Diagnostic Investigation. 2020;**32**(2):246-251

[48] Bingham C, Hodge A. Lamb mortality and clostridial disease. New Zealand Veterinary Journal. 2022;**70**(1):49-54

[49] Munday J et al. Death of a neonatal lamb due to *Clostridium perfringens* type B in New Zealand. New Zealand Veterinary Journal. 2020;**68**(4):242-246

[50] Simpson KM, Callan RJ, Van Metre DC. Clostridial abomasitis and enteritis in ruminants. The Veterinary Clinics of North America. Food Animal Practice. 2018;**34**(1):155-184

[51] Paul J. Gastrointestinal tract infections. In: Disease Causing

Microbes. Cham: Springer; 2024. DOI: 10.1007/978-3-031-28567-7_4

[52] Humphries RM, Linscott AJ. Practical guidance for clinical microbiology laboratories: Diagnosis of bacterial gastroenteritis. Clinical Microbiology Reviews. 2015;**28**(1):3-31

[53] Pawaiya RS et al. The challenges of diagnosis and control of enterotoxaemia caused by *Clostridium perfringens* in small ruminants. Advances in Microbiology. 2020;**10**(5):238-273

[54] Mileto I, Merla C, Corbella M, Gaiarsa S, Kuka A, Ghilotti S, et al. Bloodstream infection caused by *Erysipelothrix rhusiopathiae* in an immunocompetent patient. Microorganisms. 2024;**12**(5):942. DOI: 10.3390/microorganisms12050942

[55] Rostamian M, Rahmati D, Akya A. Clinical manifestations, associated diseases, diagnosis, and treatment of human infections caused by *Erysipelothrix rhusiopathiae*: A systematic review. Germs. 2022;**12**(1):16

[56] Tarasov O et al. Genome sequence of *Erysipelothrix* sp. strain poltava, isolated from acute septic erysipelas of swine in Ukraine. Microbiology Resource Announcements. 2022;**11**(8):e0043822

[57] McNeil M et al. Serotypes and Spa types of *Erysipelothrix rhusiopathiae* isolates from British pigs (1987 to 2015). Veterinary Journal. 2017;**225**:13-15

[58] Uchiyama M et al. Pathogenic characterization of *Erysipelothrix rhusiopathiae* Met-203 type SpaA strains from chronic and subacute swine erysipelas in Japan. The Journal of Veterinary Medical Science. 2017;**79**(1):18-21

[59] Ugochukwu IC et al. Erysipelas, the opportunistic zoonotic disease: History, epidemiology, pathology, and diagnosis—A review. Comparative Clinical Pathology. 2019;**28**:853-859

[60] Samrot AV et al. Leptospiral infection, pathogenesis and its diagnosis—A review. Pathogens. 2021;**10**(2):145

[61] Karpagam KB, Ganesh B. Leptospirosis: A neglected tropical zoonotic infection of public health importance-an updated review. European Journal of Clinical Microbiology & Infectious Diseases. 2020;**39**(5):835-846

[62] Bothra A et al. Cutaneous manifestations of viral outbreaks. Australasian Journal of Dermatology. 2021;**62**(1):27-36

[63] Durmaz CB, Harmankaya O, Hasman H, Gunduz A, Oktar M, Seber E et al. Acute renal failure: A common manifestation of leptospirosis. Renal Failure. 2004;**26**(6):655-661. DOI: 10.1081/JDI-200037154

[64] Adugna S. A review of bovine leptospirosis. European Journal of Applied Sciences. 2016;**8**(6):347-355

[65] Lilenbaum W, Martins G. Leptospirosis in cattle: A challenging scenario for the understanding of the epidemiology. Transboundary and Emerging Diseases. 2014;**61**:63-68

[66] Mori M et al. Reproductive disorders and leptospirosis: A case study in a mixed-species farm (cattle and swine). Veterinary Sciences. 2017;**4**(4):64

[67] Alinaitwe L et al. Cross-sectional serosurvey of Leptospira species among slaughter pigs, goats, and sheep in Uganda. PLoS Neglected Tropical Diseases. 2024;**18**(3):e0012055

[68] Hamond C et al. The role of leptospirosis in reproductive disorders in horses. Tropical Animal Health and Production. 2014;**46**:1-10

[69] Beran GW. Handbook of Zoonoses, Section A: Bacterial, Rickettsial, Chlamydial, and Mycotic Zoonoses. NY: CRC Press; 2019

[70] Richer L et al. Mouse model for sublethal *Leptospira interrogans* infection. Infection and Immunity. 2015;**83**(12):4693-4700

[71] Aymée L et al. Unconventional sites for diagnosis of leptospirosis in bovine anicteric fetuses. Animals. 2023;**13**(18):2832

[72] Evangelista KV et al. Immunoprotective properties of recombinant LigA and LigB in a hamster model of acute leptospirosis. PLoS ONE. 2017;**12**(7):e0180004

[73] Al-Orry W et al. A review of laboratory diagnosis and treatment of leptospirosis. International Journal of Pharmaceutical Sciences. 2016;**8**(12):7-13

[74] Schoen RT. Challenges in the diagnosis and treatment of Lyme disease. Current Rheumatology Reports. 2020;**22**(1):3

[75] Marques AR, Strle F, Wormser GP. Comparison of Lyme disease in the United States and Europe. Emerging Infectious Diseases. 2021;**27**(8):2017

[76] Ross Russell AL et al. Lyme disease: Diagnosis and management. Practical Neurology. 2018;**18**(6):455-464

[77] Cardenas-de la Garza JA et al. Clinical spectrum of Lyme disease. European Journal of Clinical Microbiology & Infectious Diseases. 2019;**38**(2):201-208

[78] Houston A, Macallan DC. Extrapulmonary tuberculosis. Medicine. 2014;**42**(1):18-22

[79] Admassu B, Kebede E, Shite A. Review on bovine tuberculosis. European Journal of Biological Sciences. 2015;7(4):169-185

[80] Lombard JE et al. Human-to-cattle *Mycobacterium tuberculosis* complex transmission in the United States. Frontiers in Veterinary Science. 2021;**8**:691192

[81] Alvarez J et al. Bovine tuberculosis: Within-herd transmission models to support and direct the decision-making process. Research in Veterinary Science. 2014;**97**:S61-S68

[82] Niroula N et al. Domestic pigs experimentally infected with *Mycobacterium bovis* and *Mycobacterium tuberculosis* exhibit different disease outcomes. Tuberculosis. 2022;**133**:102167

[83] Pourmahdi Borujeni M et al. Comparison of *Mycobacterium avium* subsp. paratuberculosis infection in cattle, sheep and goats in the Khuzestan Province of Iran: Results of a preliminary survey. Veterinary Medicine and Science. 2021;**7**(5):1970-1979

[84] Gelalcha BD, Zewude A, Ameni G. Tuberculosis caused by *Mycobacterium bovis* in a sheep flock colocated with a tuberculous dairy cattle herd in Central Ethiopia. Journal of Veterinary Medicine. 2019;**2019**(1):8315137

[85] Pesciaroli M et al. Tuberculosis in domestic animal species. Research in Veterinary Science. 2014;**97**:S78-S85

[86] Palmer MV et al. Tuberculosis in wild and captive deer. In: Tuberculosis, Leprosy and Mycobacterial Diseases of Man and Animals: The Many Hosts of

Mycobacteria. Wallingford UK: CABI; 2015. pp. 334-364

[87] Scanga CA, Flynn JL. Modeling tuberculosis in nonhuman primates. Cold Spring Harbor Perspectives in Medicine. 2014;**4**(12):a018564

[88] Waters WR, Palmer MV. *Mycobacterium bovis* infection of cattle and white-tailed deer: Translational research of relevance to human tuberculosis. ILAR Journal. 2015;**56**(1):26-43

[89] Allen AR, Ford T, Skuce RA. Does *Mycobacterium tuberculosis* var. *bovis* survival in the environment confound bovine tuberculosis control and eradication? A literature review. Veterinary Medicine International. 2021;**2021**(1):8812898

[90] Miller RS et al. Cross-species transmission potential between wild pigs, livestock, poultry, wildlife, and humans: Implications for disease risk management in North America. Scientific Reports. 2017;**7**(1):7821

[91] Taye H et al. Global prevalence of *Mycobacterium bovis* infections among human tuberculosis cases: Systematic review and meta-analysis. Zoonoses and Public Health. 2021;**68**(7):704-718

[92] Costa P et al. Standing of nucleic acid testing strategies in veterinary diagnosis laboratories to uncover *Mycobacterium tuberculosis* complex members. Frontiers in Molecular Biosciences. 2014;**1**:16

[93] Bruning-Fann CS et al. Use of whole-genome sequencing and evaluation of the apparent sensitivity and specificity of antemortem tuberculosis tests in the investigation of an unusual outbreak of *Mycobacterium bovis* infection in a Michigan dairy herd. Journal of the American Veterinary Medical Association. 2017;**251**(2):206-216

[94] Yee JL et al. Tuberculosis detection in nonhuman primates is enhanced by use of testing algorithms that include an interferon-γ release assay. American Journal of Veterinary Research. 2022;**83**(1):15-22

[95] Morrison LK, Willison B. Cercopithecine herpesvirus 1 (herpes B). In: Mucocutaneous Manifestations of Viral Diseases. CRC Press; 2016. pp. 206-214. eBook ISBN9780429150678

[96] Hu G et al. Herpes B virus: History, zoonotic potential, and public health implications. Biosafety and Health. 2022;**04**(04):213-219

[97] Eberle R, Jones-Engel L. Understanding primate herpesviruses. Journal of Emerging Diseases and Virology (CA, USA). Jan 31 2017;**3**(1). DOI: 10.16966/2473-1846.127

[98] Barkati S, Taher HB, Beauchamp E, Yansouni CP, Ward BJ, Libman MD. Decision tool for herpes B virus antiviral prophylaxis after macaque-related injuries in research laboratory workers. Emerging Infectious Diseases. 2019;**25**(9):e190045. DOI: 10.3201/eid2509.190045

[99] Katz D et al. Identification of unique B virus (Macacine Herpesvirus 1) epitopes of zoonotic and macaque isolates using monoclonal antibodies. PLoS ONE. 2017;**12**(8):e0182355

[100] Moghadami M. A narrative review of influenza: A seasonal and pandemic disease. Iranian Journal of Medical Sciences. 2017;**42**(1):2

[101] Gaitonde DY, Moore FC, Morgan MK. Influenza: Diagnosis and

treatment. American Family Physician. 2019;**100**(12):751-758

[102] Taubenberger JK, Kash JC, Morens DM. The 1918 influenza pandemic: 100 years of questions answered and unanswered. Science Translational Medicine. 2019;**11**(502):eaau5485

[103] Mohapatra L, Alok SGP. Alka T, Mishra D, Parida SK, Yasir M, et al. Swine flu: Current status and challenges. Rising Contagious Diseases: Basics, Management, and Treatments. NJ, USA: John Wiley & Sons, Inc.; 2024. pp. 50-65. ISBN:9781394188741. DOI: 10.1002/9781394188741.ch6

[104] Chambers TM. A brief introduction to equine influenza and equine influenza viruses. Methods in Molecular Biology (Clifton, N.J.). 2020;**2123**:355-360. DOI: 10.1007/978-1-0716-0346-8_26

[105] Veldhuis Kroeze EJ, Kuiken T. Sporadic influenza A virus infections of miscellaneous mammal species. In: Animal Influenza. 2016. pp. 557-593. DOI: 10.1002/9781118924341.ch23

[106] Frymus T et al. Influenza virus infections in cats. Viruses. 2021;**13**(8):1435

[107] Widdowson M-A, Bresee JS, Jernigan DB. The global threat of animal influenza viruses of zoonotic concern: Then and now. The Journal of Infectious Diseases. 2017;**216**(suppl. 4):S493-S498

[108] Klivleyeva NG et al. Influenza A viruses circulating in dogs: A review of the scientific literature. Open Veterinary Journal. 2022;**12**(5):676-687

[109] Margine I, Krammer F. Animal models for influenza viruses: Implications for universal vaccine development. Pathogens. 2014;**3**(4):845-874

[110] de Wit J et al. Major difference in clinical outcome and replication of a H3N1 avian influenza strain in young pullets and adult layers. Avian Pathology. 2020;**49**(3):286-295

[111] Asadi S et al. Influenza A virus is transmissible via aerosolized fomites. Nature Communications. 2020;**11**(1):4062

[112] Vemula SV et al. Current approaches for diagnosis of influenza virus infections in humans. Viruses. 2016;**8**(4):96

[113] Wobessi JNS et al. Incidence and seroprevalence of rabies virus in humans, dogs and other animal species in Africa, a systematic review and meta-analysis. One Health. 2021;**13**:100285

[114] Balcha C, Abdela N. Review of rabies preventions and control. International Journal of Public Health Science. 2017;**6**(4):343-350

[115] Beran GW. Rabies and infections by rabies-related viruses. In: Handbook of Zoonoses, Section B. CRC Press; 2017. pp. 307-357. eBook ISBN9780203752463

[116] Fisher CR, Streicker DG, Schnell MJ. The spread and evolution of rabies virus: Conquering new frontiers. Nature Reviews Microbiology. 2018;**16**(4):241-255

[117] Oliveira RN et al. Rabies virus diversification in aerial and terrestrial mammals. Genetics and Molecular Biology. 2020;**43**:e20190370

[118] Castelo-Branco D et al. Role of Brazilian bats in the epidemiological cycle of potentially zoonotic pathogens. Microbial Pathogenesis. 2023;**177**:106032

[119] Dutta TK. Rabies: An overview. International Journal of Advanced Medical and Health Research. 2014;**1**(2):39-44

[120] Ashwini MA, Pattanaik A, Mani RS. Recent updates on laboratory diagnosis of rabies. Indian Journal of Medical Research. 1 Jan 2024;**159**(1):48-61. DOI: 10.4103/ijmr.ijmr_131_23. Epub 2024 Mar 4

[121] Rasolonjatovo FS et al. Enabling animal rabies diagnostic in low-access areas: Sensitivity and specificity of a molecular diagnostic test from cerebral tissue dried on filter paper. PLoS Neglected Tropical Diseases. 2020;**14**(3):e0008116

[122] Torquato RBC et al. Detection of rabies virus antigen by the indirect rapid immunohistochemistry test in equines and comparisons with other diagnostic techniques. Zoonoses and Public Health. 2020;**67**(6):651-657

[123] Zandi M et al. Biosensor as an alternative diagnostic method for rabies virus detection: A literature review. Biotechnology and Applied Biochemistry. 2022;**69**(4):1348-1353

[124] Freuling CM, van der Westhuizen J, Khaiseb S, Tenzin T, Müller T. From field tests to molecular tools-evaluating diagnostic tests to improve rabies surveillance in Namibia. Viruses. 2023;**15**(2):371. DOI: 10.3390/v15020371

[125] Nguyen P-Y et al. Reemergence of human monkeypox and declining population immunity in the context of urbanization, Nigeria, 2017-2020. Emerging Infectious Diseases. 2021;**27**(4):1007

[126] Soheili M et al. Monkeypox: Virology, pathophysiology, clinical characteristics, epidemiology, vaccines, diagnosis, and treatments. Journal of Pharmacy & Pharmaceutical Sciences. 2022;**25**:297-322

[127] Petersen E et al. Human Monkeypox: Epidemiologic and clinical characteristics, diagnosis, and prevention. Infectious Disease Clinics of North America. 2019;**33**(4):1027-1043

[128] Martín-Delgado MC et al. Monkeypox in humans: A new outbreak. Revista Española de Quimioterapia. 2022;**35**(6):509

[129] Devaux CA et al. Infectious disease risk across the growing human-non human primate interface: A review of the evidence. Frontiers in Public Health. 2019;7:305

[130] Schmitt A, Mätz-Rensing K, Kaup F-J. Non-human primate models of orthopoxvirus infections. Veterinary Sciences. 2014;**1**(1):40-62

[131] Thèves C, Crubézy E, Biagini P. History of smallpox and its spread in human populations. In: Paleomicrobiology of Humans. 2016. pp. 161-172. DOI: 10.1128/9781555819170.ch16

[132] Shchelkunova GA, Shchelkunov SN. Smallpox, Monkeypox and other human orthopoxvirus infections. Viruses. 2022;**15**(1):103. DOI: 10.3390/v15010103

[133] Altindis M, Puca E, Shapo L. Diagnosis of monkeypox virus—An overview. Travel Medicine and Infectious Disease. 2022;**50**:102459

[134] Llorente F. West Nile Virus Infection. Pathogens. 2023;**12**:151. DOI: 10.3390/pathogens12020151

[135] Chianese A, Stelitano D, Astorri R, Serretiello E, Della Rocca MT, Melardo C, et al. West Nile virus: An overview of

current information. Translational Medicine Reports. 2019;**3**(1). DOI: 10.4081/tmr.8145

[136] Ziegler U, Santos PD, Groschup MH, Hattendorf C, Eiden M, Höper D, et al. West Nile virus epidemic in Germany triggered by epizootic emergence, 2019. Viruses. 2020;**12**(4):448. DOI: 10.3390/v12040448

[137] Schwarz ER, Long MT. Comparison of West Nile virus disease in humans and horses: Exploiting similarities for enhancing syndromic surveillance. Viruses. 2023;**15**(6):1230. DOI: 10.3390/v15061230

[138] Staji H et al. The first study of West Nile virus in feral pigeons (*Columba livia domestica*) using conventional reverse transcriptase PCR in Semnan and Khorasane-Razavi Provinces, Northeast of Iran. Journal of Arthropod-Borne Diseases. 2021;**15**(1):136-142

[139] Schvartz G et al. Molecular characterization of the re-emerging West Nile virus in avian species and equids in Israel, 2018, and pathological description of the disease. Parasites & Vectors. 2020;**13**(1):528

[140] Nwanosike H et al. Protocol of detection of West Nile virus in clinical samples. In: Bai F, editor. West Nile Virus: Methods and Protocols. New York, NY: Springer US; 2023. pp. 119-125

[141] Gómez-Vicente E et al. Comparative evaluation of chemiluminescent immunoassay and enzyme-linked immunosorbent assays for the diagnosis of West Nile virus infections. APMIS. 2022;**130**(4):215-220

Section 2

Vector-Borne Diseases

Chapter 3

Arthropods of Veterinary Importance

Jasmin Omeragić, Naida Kapo, Vedad Škapur, Šejla Goletić, Adis Softić, Ermin Šaljić and Teufik Goletić

Abstract

Arthropods are a highly diverse group of invertebrates, found in almost every habitat and constituting more than 80% of all recognized animal species. Their diversity is evident in the numerous roles they fulfill in ecosystems, including crucial functions like pollination, decomposing organic matter, and regulating pest populations. Despite their importance in maintaining ecological balance, certain arthropods can become pests in agriculture and storage, leading to crop losses and contamination of stored products. Additionally, some arthropods, such as mosquitoes, ticks, and fleas, transmit microorganisms such as bacteria, viruses, and parasites, resulting in diseases in humans and animals. Their role as vectors of pathogens is a vital research area in veterinary medicine, focusing on understanding disease transmission mechanisms and developing control strategies. Therefore, this chapter emphasizes the importance of arthropod diversity in the veterinary context and highlights various arthropod species and the pathogens they transmit.

Keywords: arthropods, importance, diversity, animals, diseases

1. Introduction

Arthropods constitute an incredibly diverse group of invertebrates, inhabiting nearly all known habitats and comprising over 80% of all known animal species [1]. The number of arthropod species exceeds the total number of all other animals on Earth, with approximately 5–10 million described species [2]. These invertebrates have significant importance in nearly all biological communities and ecosystems [3]. While many arthropods typically avoid direct contact with humans and animals, certain species become significant when we consider them as biological vectors of pathogens. Some, like flies, can act as passive carriers of pathogens. Others are ectoparasites like lice, mites and ticks, or fleas, thereby transmitting pathogens to humans and animals [4].

Given the diverse species of arthropods and the various lifestyles they demonstrate, only a small number have developed the ability to live at the expense of other animals, known as parasitism. The host offers various resources to parasites, such as food (blood, lymph, body secretions, skin debris, hair, feathers) and a suitable living environment, providing warmth, moisture, and protection. When a parasite depends on a host and its resources for its life or part of its life cycle, it is called obligatory parasitism. Obligatory parasites can spend varying amounts of time on or in the host, with some living in a constant relationship with the host. They often spread between hosts through direct contact. In contrast, facultative parasites may temporarily feed on or live on a host, but they are not dependent on it for survival. Most parasitic arthropods have only occasional contact with the host, spending the majority of their life cycles freely. Their resources depend on the host only during certain life stages [5].

Both types of interactions cause harm to the host, though they do not directly result in death. The extent of harm inflicted by a parasite can vary, sometimes becoming evident only in specific circumstances, such as when the host is in poor health or when the level of infection is high. The damage caused by arthropods can be defined practically through factors, such as compromised condition, mobility, or growth of the host.

2. Arthropods relevant to veterinary medicine

2.1 Ticks (Ixodidae, Argasidae)

Ticks, classified within the phylum Arthropoda, class Arachnida, subclass Acari, order Parasitiformes, and suborder Ixodida, include three main families: Ixodidae (hard ticks) (**Figure 1**), Argasidae (soft ticks) (**Figure 2**), and Nuttalliellidae [7–9]. Over 900 species of ticks have been classified worldwide [9]. The family Argasidae comprises a total of 193 species, primarily in two main genera: *Argas* and *Ornithodoros*. Nearly 700 species belong to the family Ixodidae, divided into main genera: *Amblyomma*, *Dermacentor*, *Haemaphysalis*, *Hyalomma*, *Ixodes,* and *Rhipicephalus* [10].

The Argasidae are generally endophilic, residing in host nests, stables, or burrows. They have a life cycle with multiple hosts and two or more nymphal stages. They rapidly take blood meals, feeding at night and typically for several minutes each time.

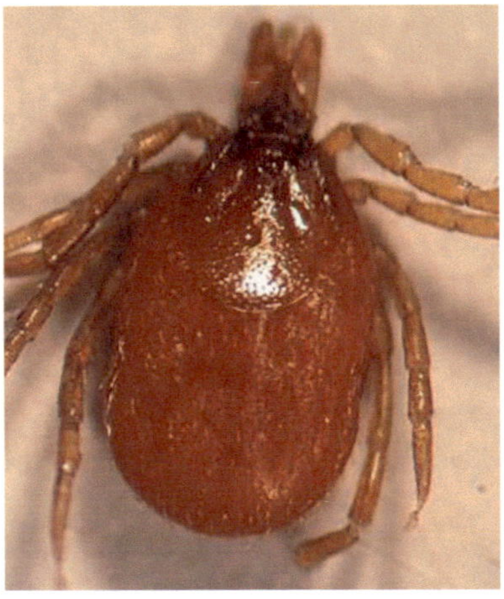

Figure 1.
Ixodes ricinus, *female [6].*

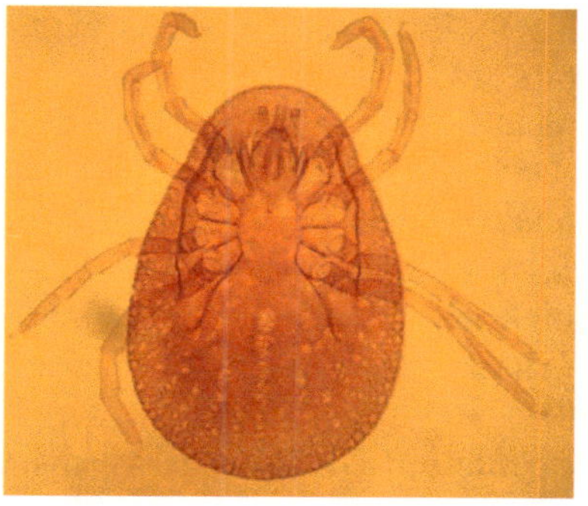

Figure 2.
Argas persicus *[6].*

The sexes are very similar; the capitulum is either ventrally located or protrudes from the anterior margin of the body in larval stages. The cuticle is smooth and leathery and there is no shield [5, 11].

Species of soft ticks of medical and veterinary significance are typically found in the genera *Argas, Ornithodoros,* and *Otobius*. They transmit various pathogens causing diseases such as tick-borne relapsing fever, which spreads worldwide through *Ornithodoros* ticks transmitting *Borrelia spirochetes* [9]. Another example is viral encephalitis transmitted by ticks found on seabirds, coastal birds, and nesting birds. Additionally, the African swine fever virus (*Asfarviridae*) is transmitted by the *Ornithodoros moubata* complex and *Ornithodoros porcinus* ticks, posing a serious threat to pigs due to high mortality rates. Spirochetosis in poultry and infections similar to anaplasmosis, caused by *Borrelia anserina* and *Aegyptianella pullorum*, are transmitted worldwide by *Argas persicus* (**Figure 2**) [5, 9].

Ixodidae are primarily exophilic ticks characterized by prolonged blood meals. Hard ticks have a life cycle involving one to three different host species, with each stage feeding on a separate host. Thus, there are one-host, two-host, and three-host hard tick life cycles. During developmental stages, ticks may remain on a specific host for each blood meal, or they may change hosts for each stage (larval, nymphal, and adult). Between feedings, they are free-living but do not feed or drink. Some ticks can survive for years without feeding. The size and body mass of ticks depend on the developmental stage, engorgement status, and species, with sizes ranging from 0.1 mm to 20 mm and from 0.04 g to 4 g in body mass [6].

Ticks are highly significant in both medical and veterinary fields, leading to considerable economic losses in global livestock farming and exerting detrimental effects on hosts through various means [11]. They parasitize a wide range of vertebrates and transmit a greater diversity of pathogenic agents more than any other group of arthropods [12]. The main losses are attributed to the ticks' ability to transmit protozoa, rickettsia, and viral pathogens, which hold great economic importance globally [13]. Tick-borne diseases in domestic animals can cause significant economic losses as a result of infertility, abortion, and mortality. These losses in turn affect livestock production characteristics, human food supply, and expenses for control measures, such as acaricide treatments [13].

Tick-borne protozoal and bacterial diseases (e.g., theileriosis and babesiosis), rickettsioses (e.g., anaplasmosis), and Q fever, as well as tick-borne dermatophilosis, constitute major health and management issues for animals in many developing countries (**Table 1**). Furthermore, most of the pathogens they transmit pose serious zoonotic threats [14].

Viruses transmitted by ticks belong to eight RNA families (*Flaviviridae*, *Reoviridae*, *Rhabdoviridae*, *Orthomyxoviridae*, *Nyamiviridae*, *Phenuiviridae*, *Nairoviridae,* and *Peribunyaviridae*) and one DNA family (*Asfarviridae*) [15]. Arboviruses, such as tick-borne encephalitis virus, West Nile virus, louping ill virus, and Powassan virus, can potentially be transmitted by various tick species, including *Dermacentor reticulatus, Ornithodoros moubata, Ixodes ricinus, Ixodes scapularis*, and *Haemaphysalis punctata* [16].

The *Nairoviridae* family contains two key viruses transmitted by ticks: Crimean-Congo hemorrhagic fever virus and the Nairobi sheep disease virus [17]. In the case of Nairobi sheep disease, mortality rates in susceptible animals exceed 90%, causing significant economic losses for production systems. Over the past two decades, epidemics of Crimean-Congo hemorrhagic fever have been recorded in many African, Asian, and European countries (**Table 1**). This virus is typically transmitted by ticks, such as *Hyalomma marginatum*, *Hyalomma lusitanicum*, *Hyalomma truncatum*, *Rhipicephalus bursa,* and *Dermacentor marginatus* [18].

Diseases caused by bacteria transmitted by ticks not only affect livestock productivity but also have zoonotic significance. Lyme disease is a prominent bacterial illness transmitted by ticks, caused by the bacterium *Borrelia burgdorferi* [19]. Ticks like *I. ricinus*, *Ixodes hexagonus*, *Ixodes pacificus*, *I. scapularis,* and *I. persulcatus* transmit these bacteria to mammalian hosts. Lyme disease affects domestic animals, showing different clinical signs (**Table 1**) [19]. Another bacterial disease transmitted by ticks is caused by the bacterium *Francisella tularensis* and is called tularemia. Different tick species like *I. ricinus*, *Dermacentor andersoni*, *Dermacentor variabilis*, *D. marginatus,* and *Amblyomma americanum* serve as vectors for *F. tularensis* [20]. These bacteria can cause illness in humans, rodents, rabbits, and occasionally sheep [20]. Besides the aforementioned, ticks such as *Haemaphysalis bispinosa* and *Ixodes holocyclus* can transmit *Coxiella burnetii*, the bacterium causing Q fever [20].

Tick-borne rickettsial diseases are caused by two groups of intracellular bacteria within the order *Rickettsiales*: bacteria belonging to the spotted fever group of the genus *Rickettsia* in the family Rickettsiaceae, and bacteria within the family Anaplasmataceae, including genera like *Anaplasma* and *Ehrlichia* [21]. Tick-borne rickettsiae can spread to new geographic regions and susceptible populations through ticks [22].

Heartwater, also known as cowdriosis, is another tick-borne rickettsial disease caused by *Ehrlichia ruminantium* (**Table 1**). Cowdriosis poses a serious threat to ruminants in sub-Saharan Africa, where a mortality rate of up to 90% has been reported [23, 24]. In dogs, *Ehrlichia canis*, *Ehrlichia ewingii*, and *Ehrlichia chaffeensis* cause Ehrlichiosis (**Table 1**). *Ehrlichia canis* is transmitted from one dog to another by the tick *Rhipicephalus sanguineus* sensu lato.

Ticks transmit numerous blood protozoa to their vertebrate hosts, with two major groups causing significant livestock diseases: theileriosis (including Tropical Theileriosis (TT) and East Coast Fever (ECF)) and babesiosis. These diseases pose substantial health and management challenges for cattle and small ruminants worldwide. The most pathogenic species are *Theileria annulata* and *Theileria parva.*

Bovine babesiosis, caused by *Babesia bovis* and *Babesia bigemina* transmitted by *Rhipicephalus microplus* and *Rhipicephalus annulatus*, and piroplasmosis in dogs caused by *Babesia canis* transmitted by *R. sanguineus* and *D. reticulatus* ticks (**Table 1**), are significant diseases affecting cattle and dogs, respectively [25].

Arthropod vectors	Diseases	Pathogens	Animals host(s)	Major geographic distribution
Ticks	Tick-borne encephalitis	*Flavivirus*	Dogs and horses	Europe and Asia
	Crimean-Congo hemorrhagic fever	*Nairovirus*	Sheep	Africa, Asia, Eastern Europe, and Middle East
	Nairobi sheep disease	*Nairovirus*	Sheep	East Africa, India, Sri Lanka, and China
	African swine fever	*Asfivirus*	Pigs	Africa, Europe, and Asia
	Lyme disease	*B. burgdorferi*	Dogs and cats	Europe, North America, and Asia
	Tularemia	*F. tularensis*	Iberian hares, wild rabbits, voles, mice, gray shrews, sheep, dogs, foxes, wolves, ticks, and river crayfish	Scandinavian countries, North America, Japan, Russia, and Western Balkan
	Anaplasmosis	*Anaplasma* spp.	Dogs, cats, horses and ruminants	Europe, America, Africa, Asia and Australia
	Heartwater (or cowdriosis)	*E. ruminantium*	Domestic and wild ruminants	Sub-Sahelian Africa and Caribbean islands
	Ehrlichiosis	*Ehrlichia canis*, *E. ewingii*, *E. chaffeensis*	Dogs	Worldwide
	Tropical theileriosis	*T. annulata*	Cattle	Europe, Asia, and Africa
	East Coast fever	*T. parva*	Cattle	Central, eastern, and southern Africa
	Babesiosis	*Babesia* spp.	Cattle, sheep, goats, dogs, cats, horses and pigs	Europe, Asia, Africa, North America, South America, and Australia
	Tick-borne ehrlichiosis	*Ehrlichia* spp.	Dogs and cats	Worldwide

Arthropod vectors	Diseases	Pathogens	Animals host(s)	Major geographic distribution
Lice	Swine pox	*Suipoxvirus*	Pigs	Worldwide
Fleas	Dipilidiosis	*D. caninum*	Domestic and wild carnivores	Worldwide
	Bartonellosis	*Bartonella* spp.	Dogs and cats	Worldwide
	Rickettsiosis	*Rickettsia* spp.	Dogs and cats	Worldwide
	Filariasis	*A. reconditum*	Domestic and wild carnivores	Worldwide
Sand Flies	Leishmaniasis	*Leishmania spp.*	Domestic and wild animals	Europe, Africa, the Americas, Asia, and Australia
	Vesicular stomatitis	*Vesiculovirus*	Equines, cattle, swine and camelids	South and North America
Biting Midges	Epizootic Hemorrhagic Disease	*Orbivirus*	Domestic and wild ruminants	North America, Australia, Asia, Africa, and Mediterranean Basin
	African Horse Sickness	*Orbivirus*	Equids	Sub-Saharan Africa, Spain, Middle East, and the Indian subcontinent
	Schmallenberg Disease	*Orthobunyavirus*	Domestic and wild ruminants	Europe and Middle East
	Bluetongue	*Orbivirus*	Domestic and wild ruminants	Worldwide

Arthropod vectors	Diseases	Pathogens	Animals host(s)	Major geographic distribution
Mosquitoes	Yellow fever	*Flavivirus*	Monkeys	South America
	Dengue	*Flavivirus*	Bats, non-human primates, birds, dogs, horses, pigs, and rodents	Europe, Africa, South America, and United States
	Rift Valley fever	*Phlebovirus*	Cattle, sheep, goats, and camels	Africa and Arabian Peninsula
	Wesselsbron disease	*Flavivirus*	Cattle and sheep	Africa
	Myxomatosis	*Leporipoxvirus*	Rabbits	Europe, Australia, South and North America
	Eastern equine encephalomyelitis	*Alphavirus*	Horses, birds, and dogs	Central, South, and North America
	Western equine encephalomyelitis	*Alphavirus*	Horses	Central, South, and North America
	Venezuelan equine encephalomyelitis	*Alphavirus*	Horses	Central, South, and North America
	Wesselsbron disease	*Flavivirus*	Livestock and wild animals	Africa and Asia
	Japanese encephalitis	*Flavivirus*	Horses and pigs	Europe, Asia, and Africa
	Chikungunya fever	*Alphavirus*	Green monkeys, baboons, and wild primates	West Africa and East/Central/South Africa
	Zika encephalitis	*Flavivirus*	Monkeys	Asia, French Polynesia and other islands in the Pacific Ocean, parts of South, Central and North America
	West Nile fever	*Flavivirus*	Horses, birds, alpaca, harbor seal, reindeer, Barbary macaque, white-tailed deer, and polar bear	Africa, the Middle East, and Europe and United States
	Dog heartworm	*Dirofilaria* spp.	Dogs, cats	Worldwide
Black Flies	Onchocerciasis	*Onchocerca* spp.,	Red deer, moose, sika deer, donkeys, cattle, horses, dogs, wolves, and wild boar	Europe, Africa, Asia, Middle East, South America, and Australia
	Vesicular stomatitis	*Vesiculovirus*	Cattle, horses, and pigs	South and North America

Arthropod vectors	Diseases	Pathogens	Animals host(s)	Major geographic distribution
Tsetse flies	Animal African trypanosomiasis (nagana)	*Trypanosoma* spp.	Domestic and wild animals	Africa
Horse flies and deer flies	Surra (livestock trypanosomiasis)	*Trypanosoma evansi*	Camels, equids, cattle, and buffaloes	Europe, Africa, Asia, Middle East, and South America
	Equine infectious anemia	Lentivirus	Horses	Worldwide
	Bovine besnoitiosis	*Besnotia besnoiti*	Ruminants	Africa, Asia, and Europe
Muscidae	Habronemiasis	Draschia *megastoma, Habronema majus*, and *H. muscae*	Donkeys, horses, mules, zebras, and dogs	Worldwide

Table 1.
Examples of arthropod-borne diseases: Importance in veterinary medicine.

DOI: http://dx.doi.org/10.5772/intechopen.1006979

2.2 Mites (Acari)

Mites have been successful in parasitizing all major vertebrate groups except for fish. Some mites act as vectors for pathogens of domestic and wild animals, while others act as intermediate hosts for animal parasites, particularly cestodes.

According to classification schemes, mites or Acari are categorized into two main groups: the superorder Parasitiformes (Anactinotrichida) and the superorder Acariformes (Actinotrichida). These groups are further subdivided into six orders: Opilioacarida (Notostigmata), Holothyrida (Tetrastigmata), Ixodida (Metastigmata), Mesostigmata (Gamasida), Trombidiformes (including Prostigmata, Actinedida, and Tarsonemida), and Sarcoptiformes (including Oribatida, Astigmata, and Endeostigmata) [8, 26]. Members of the orders Ixodida, Mesostigmata, Trombidiformes, and Sarcoptiformes are known to cause health issues in animals.

Dermanyssidae, Macronyssidae, Trombiculidae, and Laelapidae, which live on the surface of animals, often cause irritation when they bite hosts to feed on blood, lymph, or skin tissues [5, 27].

2.2.1 Dermanyssidae

2.2.1.1 Red poultry mite (Dermanyssus gallinae)

Dermanyssus gallinae (**Figure 3**), the red poultry mite (RPM), parasitizes wild and domestic birds worldwide, including chickens, ducks, pigeons, and canaries. It can also infest dogs, cats, horses, cows, and other mammals. *Dermanyssus gallinae* measures approximately 1.5 mm in length, with coloration ranging from gray to brown/red, depending on its feeding status.

During the day, it hides in cracks, emerging at night to feed on birds. Chronic or severe infestations result in skin irritation, slowed growth, reduced egg production, anemia, and death due to blood loss. Dogs exposed to *D. gallinae* around poultry houses at night may have adverse reactions to their bites, including intense itching, reduced activity during the day, and signs of depression.

Dermanyssus gallinae is an increasing epidemiological and economic problem for the poultry industry worldwide [5]. Infection rates of 80–90% have been documented

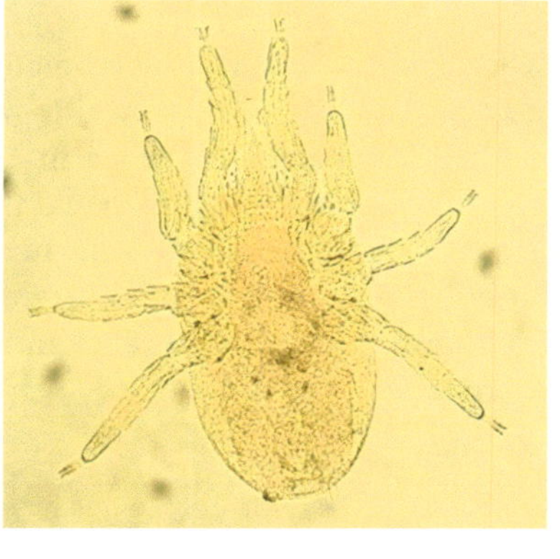

Figure 3.
Dermanyssus gallinae, *red poultry mite [6].*

in poultry birds across various countries, including the United Kingdom (UK), Italy, Serbia, Morocco, Japan, Montenegro, and the Netherlands [28].

2.2.2 Macronyssidae

Most members of the Macronyssidae family are obligatory parasites of vertebrates, originally evolving on bats and later transferring to other mammals, reptiles, and birds [29]. Some mites from the family Macronyssidae have invaded the oral mucosa of bats that feed on pollen and fruit (Phyllostomidae) [5].

2.2.3 Trombiculidae, Leeuwenhoekiidae, Walchiidae

The larvae of these families, commonly referred to as chiggers, red bugs, and berry bugs, exhibit a broad host range, including amphibians, reptiles, birds, and mammals, with humans being incidental hosts [30, 31]. These trombiculoid mite larvae often infest domestic animals, with noticeable symptoms typically arising only in cases of severe infestation or hypersensitivity reactions. Similarly to humans, animals that are incidental hosts may develop dermatitis in response to mite activity.

2.2.4 Fur mites

Fur mites are specifically adapted to live in the fur of mammals. Six groups of particular veterinary interest are the cheyletoid families Cheyletidae and Myobiidae, as well as the astigmatid families Listrophoridae, Atopomelidae, Chirodiscidae, and Myocoptidae.

2.2.4.1 Cheyletidae

Parasitic Cheyletidae mites inhabit the hair of domestic cats, dogs, rabbits, and various wild mammals and birds, feeding on lymph and tissue fluids by piercing the epidermis [32]. Transmission usually occurs through direct contact with infected animals, including transmission from mother to offspring during nursing. *Cheyletiella* mites are often associated with fleas in cats and dogs (*Ctenocephalides* spp.) and can also be transmitted through these ectoparasites.

2.2.4.2 Myobiidae

Members of the family Myobiidae are obligatory parasites of rodents, bats, insectivores, and certain marsupials. The mites move along the hairs up and down and remain attached to the hair while feeding on epidermal fluids. Their chelicerae are long and pointed, adapted for piercing thin epidermal tissues to suck extracellular fluid. Most species cause little obvious discomfort or harm to their hosts, even when the number of mites is high. Exceptions of veterinary interest include several species of *Myobia* and *Radfordia* that commonly infest rats and mice, often causing mild to severe dermatitis and scaling in laboratory rodents [5].

2.2.4.3 Listrophoridae

Listrophorid mites are obligatory parasites of rodents, rabbits, carnivores, and other mammalian hosts [5]. They predominantly feed on sebaceous secretions, typically causing minor harm, even when present in large numbers. However, exceptions occur in rodents and rabbits, particularly in captive or overcrowded conditions. In such cases, severe infestations can lead to dermatitis, itching, and hair loss.

2.2.5 Mange mites

The species causing mange in animals, including livestock, poultry, and pets belong to the families Epidermoptidae, Dermationidae, Knemidokoptidae, Laminosioptidae, Demodecidae, Psorergatidae, Sarcoptidae, Psoroptidae, Harpirhynchidae, and Hypoderatidae. The prevalence of mange mite infestation is affected by various factors including age, body condition, breed, and environmental conditions [33, 34].

2.2.5.1 Epidermoptidae and Dermationidae

Mites of the families Epidermoptidae and Dermationidae are permanent parasites living on or in the skin of birds (Acari: Analgoidea) [35]. Several species within these families have been reported to cause discomfort and injuries to infected birds. They reside on the skin or in feather follicles, causing itching, crusty dermatitis, and other skin lesions.

2.2.5.2 Knemidokoptidae

Knemidokoptidae mites resemble sarcoptid mites but have short legs without pretarsi or long setae, and lack dorsal triangular spines (**Figure 4**). Species of veterinary significance that infest the feather follicles and skin of wild and domestic birds worldwide include *Knemidokoptes mutans*, *Neocnemidocoptes gallinae*, *K. pilae*, and *K. jamaicensis* [5].

2.2.5.3 Demodecidae

Infestation by Demodecidae mites is termed demodicosis, while cases exhibiting clinical symptoms are referred to as demodectic mange [36]. These mites are host-specific and typically localize within hair follicles or dermal glands, including sebaceous glands, modified sebaceous glands, modified sweat glands, and mixed sebaceous-sweat glands. Several species penetrate the skin to create epidermal

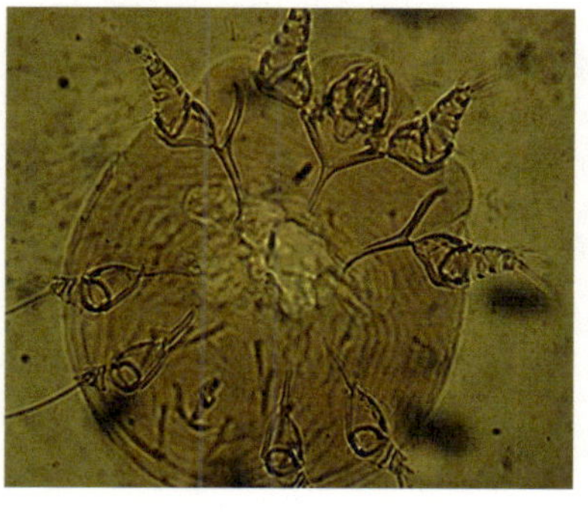

Figure 4.
Knemidocoptes *spp. [6].*

burrows, and other species from the family Demodecidae invade the oral tissues of hosts, infecting the oral epithelium, tongue, and esophagus [37].

Demodectic mange is common in domestic and wild animals. It is relatively uncommon in cats and horses. *Demodex canis* (**Figure 5**) inhabits hair follicles and sebaceous glands of dogs worldwide, along with two other species, *Demodex injai* and *Demodex cornei*. *Demodex injai* primarily appears in sebaceous glands and ducts, while *D. cornei* inhabits the keratinized layer of the epidermis. Lesions attributed to *Demodex cati* and *Demodex gatoi* sometimes develop in cats, typically presenting as the squamous form of demodicosis. In livestock, demodicosis is caused by *Demodex bovis* and *Demodex tauri*. Demodicosis in goats, caused by *Demodex caprae*, is most frequently observed in young animals, pregnant, and lactating goats [5, 38].

2.2.5.4 Sarcoptidae

The Sarcoptidae family encompasses three significant genera that infest both domestic and wild animals: *Sarcoptes*, *Notoedres*, and *Trixacarus*. Sarcoptic mites causing mange in animals are morphologically indistinguishable from the mite that causes scabies in humans, *Sarcoptes scabiei* [5].

Almost all domestic animals, except cats and guinea pigs, are susceptible to infestations of *S. scabiei*. Certain wild mammal groups, including members of the families Canidae, Procyonidae, and Cervidae, are particularly prone to sarcoptic mange caused by *S. scabiei* [38]. The most severe cases are reported in foxes during the winter months.

2.2.5.5 Notoedres species

Notoedres mites cause severe dermatitis in small mammals, felids, and procyonids and occasionally affect humans as a zoonosis [5, 39]. They are cutaneous parasites that typically burrow into the horn-like layer of the skin, causing inflammation, crusted lesions, and hair loss known as notoedric mange. Common hosts include cats (*Notoedres cati*) (**Figure 6**), rats (*Notoedres muris*), squirrels (*Notoedres centrifera*), rabbits, and bats. *Notoedres* species are occasionally reported as parasites of dogs, foxes, civets, lorises (primates), koalas, bandicoots (marsupials), hamsters, and hedgehogs [39].

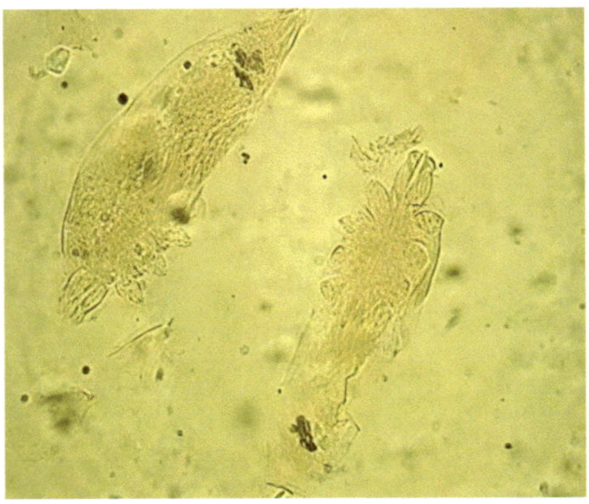

Figure 5.
Demodex canis *[6]*.

DOI: http://dx.doi.org/10.5772/intechopen.1006979

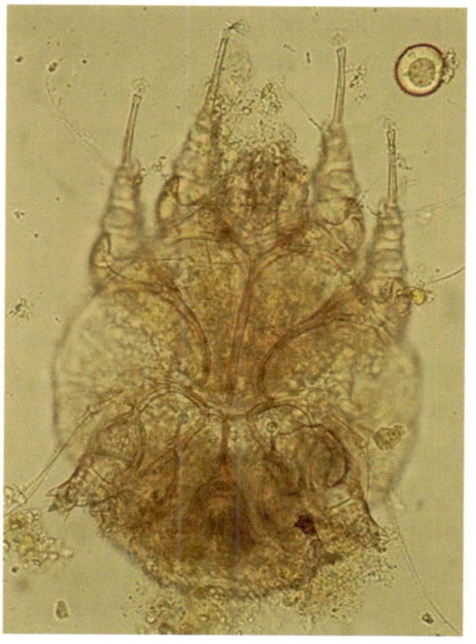

Figure 6.
Notoedres cati *[6].*

2.2.5.6 Psoroptidae

Mites from the family Psoroptidae are mammalian ectoparasites commonly known as mange mites. All developmental stages occur in the host. They do not penetrate the epidermis but rather live on the skin surface. Feeding often results in inflammation, itching, and crust formation. Scratching and rubbing often cause the host's hair to tangle and severely damage the skin [5].

Psoroptid mange mites of veterinary interest primarily parasitize Artiodactyla, Perissodactyla, and Carnivora. They are also found in certain marsupials, insectivores, and primates. *Psoroptes* mites attack cattle, sheep, goats, horses, and rabbits; *Chorioptes* mites are mainly problematic in cattle; *Otodectes* mites cause problems in cats and dogs; while *Caparinia* mites infest hedgehogs.

Chorioptic mange, caused by *Chorioptes bovis*, occurs in domestic ungulates such as cattle, sheep, goats, and horses. As a group, chorioptic mites are primarily parasites of herbivores (Artiodactyla, Perissodactyla, and Lagomorpha), including llamas, guanacos, alpacas, and rabbits [40].

2.2.5.7 Ear mites

Several species of mites infest the ears of domestic and wild animals, with the most common belonging to the families Psoroptidae, Trombiculidae, and Raillietidae.

Sweatman [41] identified five distinct species of the genus *Psoroptes* based on morphological traits, host specificity, and body localization: *Psoroptes cuniculi*, *Psoroptes cervinus*, *Psoroptes natalensis*, *Psoroptes equi*, and *Psoroptes ovis*. Localization on the host was proposed as a significant taxonomic criterion, distinguishing between "ear mites," found in the ear canal, and "body mites," occurring elsewhere on the body [41, 42].

Psoroptes ovis causes lesions in laboratory rabbits and in commercial rabbitries, known as psoroptic otocariasis. This cosmopolitan mite also infests the ears of sheep, goats, horses, deer, and guinea pigs, causing crusts, discharge, ear scratching, and head shaking. Severe infestations can spread to the face, neck, and legs.

Otodectes cynotis, ear mite, causes otodectic mange in cats and dogs and also affects other carnivores like foxes, ferrets, squirrels, and raccoons worldwide. Cattle and goat ear mites, *Raillietia* spp., are the only known mesostigmatid mites that inhabit the ear canals of domestic animals [5, 43].

2.3 Lice (Phthiraptera)

Lice pose a threat to humans, pets, and livestock by sucking blood or chewing and transmitting pathogens. The Phthiraptera is divided into sucking lice, which are obligate blood-feeding ectoparasites of mammals, and chewing lice, which primarily feed on feathers, fur, skin, or skin products. Sucking lice are more significant in pathogen transmission due to their blood-feeding habits. Phthiraptera are divided into four suborders: Anoplura, Amblycera, Ischnocera, and Rhynchophthirina. Previous classifications treated Anoplura and Mallophaga as separate orders, with Amblycera, Ischnocera, and Rhynchophthirina all included within Mallophaga.

Relatively few species of lice of veterinary significance transmit pathogens. Lice in cattle, sheep, and goats cause economic problems worldwide. These animals are typically parasitized by one species each of Haematopinus, Linognathus, Solenopotes, and Bovicola. Horses, donkeys, pigs, goats, and sheep are all parasitized by one or more species of lice [5].

In domestic and wild cats, one species of chewing louse parasitizes (*Felicola subrostrata*), while dogs have two species of chewing lice and one species of sucking louse (*Heterodoxus spiniger*, *Trichodectes canis*, and *Linognathus setosus*). Both types of lice found in dogs, the dog louse (*T. canis*) and the dog sucking louse (*L. setosus*), parasitize domestic dogs and related wild canids (coyotes, foxes, and wolves). Another species of chewing louse, *H. spiniger*, originated in Australasia from lice that parasitized marsupials and apparently transferred to dingoes. It now parasitizes various canids of other carnivores worldwide [5, 44].

Lice infestation, presumed to be caused by their diet and movement on the host, can be extremely irritating. The host may develop dermatitis, allergic reactions, or secondary infections contributing to itching. Furthermore, licking can lead to the formation of hairballs in the stomach, especially in cats and calves. Infestations of sucking lice can compromise the host's vitality, leading to anemia, abortion, and death.

Only a small number of pathogens transmitted to domestic animals via lice are recognized, with notable examples being the swine pox virus and bacterial agents such as *Mycoplasma muris* and *Mycoplasma coccoides* causing murine mycoplasma infection (**Table 1**). Additionally, *Mycoplasma suis*, which causes acute febrile illness in pigs, is reported to be transmitted via pig lice according to some researchers. Swinepox, a significant viral illness in pigs primarily affects young piglets in unsanitary conditions. The pig louse *Haematopinus suis* serves as the main mechanical vector for transmission [45]. Other pathogens have been identified in different species of lice, however, there is no current evidence to suggest that lice act as vectors for these organisms [46].

Lice in pets are most noticeable in sick, malnourished hosts that often cannot groom themselves or in very young or old animals. Additionally, the dog louse serves as an intermediate host for the double tapeworm (*Dipylidium caninum*). Lice become infected by ingesting viable *D. caninum* eggs from the host's dry feces, where the tapeworm develops into a cysticercoid and remains dormant until the louse is ingested by a dog during grooming. Once in the dog's intestine, the cysticercoid matures into an adult worm [47].

The sucking louse of dogs (*L. setosus*) is widespread worldwide. This louse often appears primarily on the neck, shoulders, under the collar, and mostly on long-haired breeds of dogs. Lice can cause irritation, resulting in insomnia, nervousness, chewing, and scratching. This species has been found to host immature forms of the filarial nematode *Acanthocheilonema reconditum*, which infects dogs.

2.4 Fleas (Siphonaptera)

Fleas are morphologically unique ectoparasites that are easily distinguished from other arthropods. Currently, about 2500 species and subspecies of fleas have been described, classified into 18 families and 220 genera [48]. Most fleas of medical or veterinary significance belong to the family Pulicidae, while other important fleas belong to the families Tungidae, Ceratophyllidae, Leptopsyllidae, or Vermipsyllidae [49].

2.4.1 Dog flea (Ctenocephalides canis)

Ctenocephalides felis is the predominant flea species affecting dogs and cats across Europe and the United States [49], whereas *Ctenocephalides canis* (**Figure 7**) is primarily associated with dogs and has a more limited geographical range [50]. The prevalence of this flea species on domestic dogs has decreased in many parts of the world. Instead, the cat flea has become the predominant flea species on domestic dogs in most regions. There is no definitive explanation for this shift; cat fleas may outcompete dog fleas, which may be affected by modern pesticides. However, dog fleas are still found globally and remain prevalent in dogs in certain areas. *Ctenocephalides canis* also infests wild canids such as foxes, where they are relatively common.

2.4.2 Cat flea (Ctenocephalides felis)

Ctenocephalides felis (**Figure 8**) holds significant importance as an ectoparasite affecting dogs, cats and other domestic animals globally, given its widespread presence. It serves a dual role as both an infesting organism and a disease vector, resulting in economic losses and the development of resistance to conventional insecticides [51, 52]. It also parasitizes wild mammals such as opossums and raccoons, with some strains of the cat flea appearing to have adapted to ungulates, such as horses or goats. Female cat fleas produce prolific numbers of fertile eggs, laying up to about 25 per day over a month under ideal conditions, leading to rapid population growth. The cat

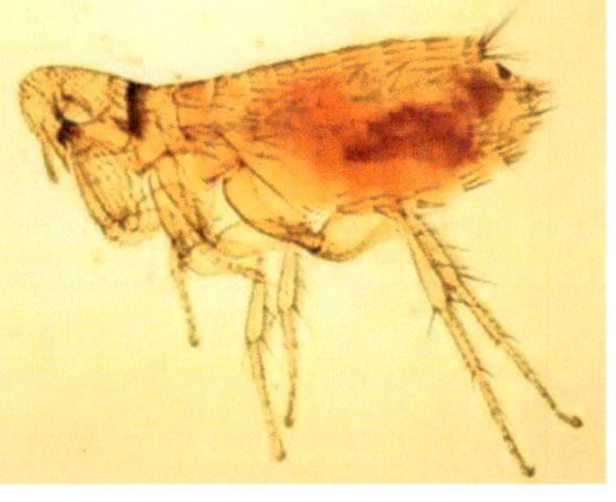

Figure 7.
Ctenocephalides canis *[6].*

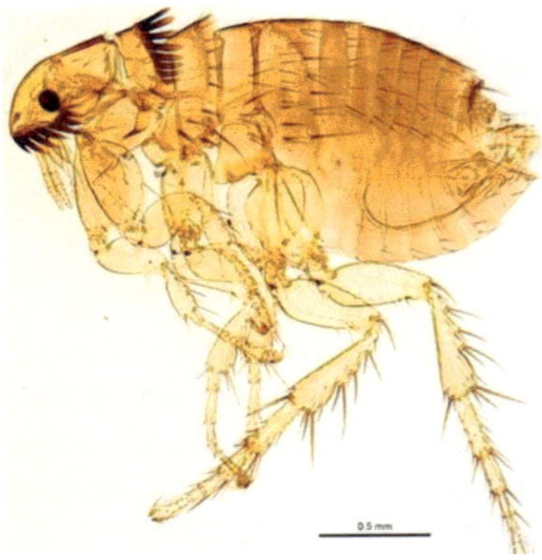

Figure 8.
Ctenocephalides felis *[6]*.

flea can vector multiple zoonotic organisms, including *Bartonella* spp., *Dipylidium caninum*, and *Rickettsia* spp. (**Table 1**).

Many fleas associated with domestic animals are primarily bothersome due to their bites, but they can also cause dermatitis with allergic reactions and anemia. Other fleas, such as sticktight and chigoes, embed deeply into the tissues of mammals or birds, causing local inflammation and other problems. Some flea species act as intermediaries for helminths that parasitize domestic animals, while others transmit pathogens such as viruses and trypanosomes to their hosts.

Other fleas that irritate domestic mammals include *Pulex simulans*, the human flea (*Pulex irritans*), and the sticktight flea (*Echidnophaga gallinacea*), which can parasitize both cats and dogs. *Pulex simplex* can be found on dogs and pigs, while *E. gallinacea* is found in a variety of mammals.

The main intermediate hosts for *Dipylidium caninum* are cat fleas and dog fleas, with the human flea also able to serve in that role. *Dipylidium caninum* is distributed worldwide, occurring on all continents (with the exception of Antarctica) (**Table 1**). In tropical Africa, the pig flea (*Echidnophaga larina*) is sometimes responsible for infestations in household dogs.

Two species of tapeworms that commonly affect rats and mice as adult individuals are the rat tapeworm (*Hymenolepis diminuta*) and the dwarf tapeworm (*Rodentolepis nana*).

The nematode *Acanthocheilonema reconditum*, responsible for a relatively mild form of filariasis in dogs, jackals, and hyenas worldwide, has been found in several flea species. Cat fleas and dog fleas are considered the main vectors, with transmission likely occurring when carnivores ingest infected fleas while grooming.

2.5 Phlebotomine sand flies

The Psychodidae family comprises approximately 3400 species distributed among six existing subfamilies and one extinct subfamily. Among these, the subfamily Phlebotominae is of significant medical and veterinary interest [5]. They have a wide host range and are proven or suspected vectors of several pathogens, including leishmaniasis, bartonellosis, and sand fly fevers [53]. The taxonomy of the subfamily Phlebotominae began in 1786 and gained significant attention in the early twentieth century when some of its species were linked to the transmission of leishmaniasis agents. Currently, this group encompasses 1060 described species and subspecies worldwide [54, 55].

The bacterial disease bartonellosis in humans is transmitted by several species of Phlebotominae [56]. However, members of Phlebotominae can also cause damage to livestock, pets, and wildlife in areas where they are abundant. Additionally, they can transmit *Leishmania* to dogs and cats and may also play a role in the transmission of vesicular stomatitis virus among livestock (**Table 1**).

Among the 31 *Leishmania* species that infect humans and animals worldwide, *Leishmania infantum* is the only autochthonous species in Europe, while *Leishmania tropica* and *Leishmania donovani* sensu stricto appear sporadically and locally [57, 58]. Dogs are the main domestic reservoir of *L. infantum* and the most susceptible host species, while humans are considered accidental hosts.

2.6 Biting midges (Ceratopogonidae)

Biting midge species within the Diptera family Ceratopogonidae can pose a significant nuisance to both livestock and humans, particularly in certain regions and seasons.

The Ceratopogonidae family is a diverse, abundant, and broadly distributed group. They are divided into four subfamilies: Leptoconopinae, Forcipomyiinae, Dasyheleinae, and Ceratopogoninae. Except for Dasyheleinae, species in each subfamily feed on the blood of vertebrates. Species in only four genera are known for their attacks on humans and other animals. The most significant genus in this regard is *Culicoides*.

The *Culicoides obsoletus* complex (**Figure 9**) and *Culicoides pulicaris* complex are increasingly associated with the transmission of Bluetongue virus (BTV) in the Palearctic region. The *Culicoides imicola* complex includes 10 morphological species. This complex is limited to the Old World, where it plays an important role in the transmission of viruses causing African horse sickness and BT.

2.6.1 Epizootic hemorrhagic disease

Epizootic hemorrhagic disease (EHD) is an arthropod-transmitted viral illness of wild and domestic ruminants [59]. Biting midges of the genus *Culicoides* are the only known vectors of the EHD virus. EHDV is a member of the *Reoviridae* family,

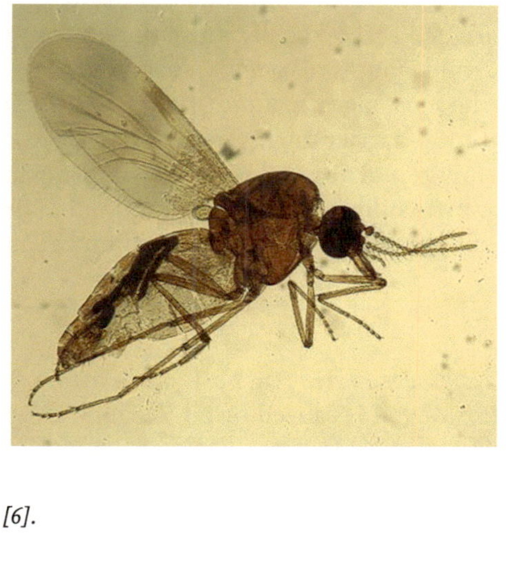

Figure 9.
Culicoides obsoletus, *imago [6].*

Orbivirus genus. Currently, there are seven recognized serotypes of EHDV, with the Ibaraki virus representing serotype 2 (EHDV-2) and causing sporadic outbreaks in cattle in Asia. The global distribution and epidemiology of BTV and EHDV infections are similar.

Most natural and experimental EHDV infections in livestock, except for Ibaraki virus, are subclinical. However, outbreaks of EHD have been documented in cattle across the Mediterranean Basin, Reunion Island, South Africa, and other regions (**Table 1**) [60–63]. Certain strains of EHDV, notably Ibaraki virus (EHDV-2) and newly identified strains of EHDV-2, EHDV-6, and EHDV-7, have demonstrated increased virulence in cattle in multiple countries. Nevertheless, the molecular mechanisms underlying EHDV virulence remain unclear, as strains of the same serotypes typically do not cause significant disease in cattle in other endemic regions.

2.6.2 African horse sickness

African horse sickness (AHS) is a fatal viral disease affecting horses, donkeys, and mules. The etiological agent of AHS is a species in the *Orbivirus* genus (*Reoviridae*), closely related to viruses causing BT disease and EHD (**Table 1**). Nine serotypes of AHS have been recognized, all of which occur in eastern and southern Africa. Only serotypes 4 and 9 appear in West Africa and along the Mediterranean coast. The virus can be transmitted 12 to 13 days after an infected blood meal. Four clinical forms of AHS are recognized: pulmonary (peracute), cardiac (subacute), mixed pulmonary-cardiac (acute), and fever.

The primary vectors of the AHS virus are *Culicoides* species, with *C. imicola* predominantly responsible in Africa and the Middle East, while *Culicoides bolitinos* plays a secondary role. Furthermore, it is assumed that the camel tick (*Hyalomma dromedarii*) plays a secondary role as a vector for AHS.

2.6.3 Schmallenberg disease

Schmallenberg virus (SBV) is a member of the Orthobunyavirus genus within the Peribunyaviridae family (**Table 1**). It has been demonstrated that SBV is transmitted via *C. obsoletus*, *Culicoides scoticus*, and *Culicoides punctatus* [63]. While originally identified in sheep, goats, and cattle, subsequent epidemiological studies have linked SBV to wild ruminants including deer, mouflon, and bison. In adult ruminants, SBV infection often goes unnoticed as it typically presents as asymptomatic. However, in cases of acute infection, mild symptoms such as fever, diarrhea, or decreased milk production may occur. The most significant impact of SBV infection occurs when the virus crosses the placental barrier during a critical period of pregnancy. This can result in severe developmental abnormalities in offspring, including joint stiffness, tendon shortening, torticollis, hydranencephaly, and hydrocephalus, as well as stillbirths, premature delivery, and mummification of embryos and fetuses.

2.6.4 Bluetongue

BT is a significant viral disease affecting both domestic and wild ruminants, with notable economic implications. It is caused by BTV, which belongs to the *Orbivirus* genus within the *Reoviridae* family. To date, 28 serotypes of BTV have been identified globally, with 23 of these serotypes reported in India [64]. BTV is primarily transmitted by *Culicoides* midges and can lead to clinical disease in species, such as sheep, white-tailed deer, pronghorn antelope, and bighorn sheep. While cattle, goats, and camelids may also be affected, they often exhibit subclinical manifestations of the disease.

Ruminants infected with BTV often exhibit noticeable symptoms such as lameness, reluctance to move, and weight loss, primarily due to inflammation in muscles and hooves. The disease derives its name from the occasional bluish or blue-red discoloration observed on the oral mucosa and tongue, resulting from cyanosis. In pregnant females, BTV infection can lead to stillbirths and fetal malformations [65].

2.7 Black flies (Simuliidae)

Black flies can be significant pests of humans, domestic animals, and wildlife, affecting various aspects of life. They are widespread worldwide, except in Antarctica and some island regions and inhabit elevational ranges from below sea level to at least 5000 meters above sea level [66, 67].

More than 2200 species of black flies have been described worldwide [67]. The subfamily Simuliinae is divided into two tribes, the Prosimuliini and the Simuliini, the latter including the majority of pest species [68]. Black flies are significant bloodsucking vectors known for transmitting filarial nematodes, trypanosomes, haemosporidian parasites, and vesicular stomatitis viruses (**Table 1**) [69].

Deaths of birds and livestock result from the overwhelming attacks of large numbers of black flies, causing panic, injuries, and even suffocation due to airway blockage and respiratory infections. Continuous attacks by black flies on poorly protected areas such as the ears, neck, and ventral midline can lead to restless behavior, weight loss, imbalanced nutrition in young animals, dermatitis, epidermal necrosis, and potentially stress-related diseases like pneumonia.

2.8 Mosquitoes (Culicidae)

The Culicidae family, known as mosquitoes, encompasses approximately 3587 species classified into the subfamilies Anophelinae and Culicinae. Anophelines carry characteristic floating eggs, their larvae lack respiratory siphons, and adults have elongated palps in both sexes.

There are 41 genera of mosquitoes, with 38 belonging to the subfamily Culicinae. Three important groups of mosquito species worldwide are the *Anopheles gambiae* and *Culex pipiens* complexes, and the subgenus *Aedes*, *Stegomyia* (**Figure 10**). They are vectors of several pathogens, including protozoa such as *Plasmodium* spp. nematodes like filariae, and viruses such as dengue, chikungunya, West Nile, and Zika [5].

Over 620 arboviruses are associated with arthropods, nearly half with mosquitoes, and about 100 infect humans and animals. "Arbovirus" means "arthropod-borne virus" and lacks formal taxonomic significance. Key mosquito-borne viruses affecting humans include *Alphavirus* (*Togaviridae*), *Flavivirus* (*Flaviviridae*), *Orthobunyavirus*, and *Phlebovirus* (*Bunyaviridae*).

Aedes aegypti, known as the yellow fever mosquito, spreads across tropical and subtropical areas worldwide and is the vector of dengue virus, yellow fever, Chikungunya, and Zika viruses. *Aedes albopictus*, known as the Asian tiger mosquito, oviposits in natural containers like tree holes, water-holding containers, and different types of plastic containers where the larvae develop and transmit dengue, Chikungunya, and Zika viruses. Initially restricted to Asia, where it occurs in rural areas of tropical and subtropical regions.

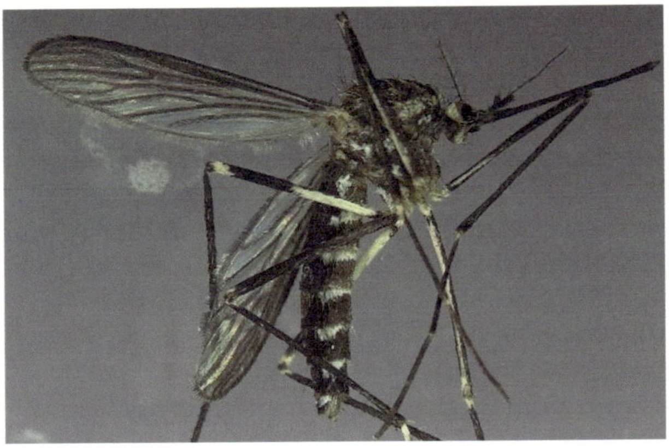

Figure 10.
Aedes *spp. [6].*

2.8.1 Eastern equine encephalitis (EEE)

Eastern equine encephalitis virus (EEEV) is a mosquito-borne virus belonging to the *Alphavirus* genus, Togaviridae family, and is closely related to Western equine encephalitis virus and Venezuelan equine encephalitis virus [70]. This virus is a significant cause of mortality in horses and other hoofed animals, cage-reared pheasants, and grouse. It occurs in endemic areas of the United States (**Table 1**). Horses quickly succumb to infection after a short incubation period of 2–5 days. They exhibit unusual behavior and high fever, then collapse and fall into a coma before death. In flocks of pheasants, one infected bird is often pecked by other birds, thereby transmitting the virus directly to healthy birds without mosquito bites. EEE virus infection has been reported in young dogs and pigs.

2.8.2 Western equine encephalitis virus (WEE)

Western Equine Encephalitis Virus (WEEV) is a mosquito-borne *Alphavirus* (family *Togaviridae*) that causes severe neurological disease in humans and equids (**Table 1**) [71]. Similar to the EEE virus, the primary epizootic host of significance for the WEE virus is the horse. Immunization has reduced the frequency of cases in horses for both EEE and WEE viruses.

2.8.3 Japanese encephalitis (JE)

Japanese encephalitis virus (JEV) is a positive-sense single-stranded RNA virus of the *Flavivirus* genus that is spread by *Culex* mosquitos (**Table 1**) [72]. Encephalitis occurs in wide areas of Asia, including Malaysia and Indonesia. The JEV causes acute infection in horses and pigs. It poses a particular economic problem due to the importance of pigs as a source of food and marketable goods in rural Asia [5].

2.8.4 Rift Valley fever (RVF)

Rift Valley Fever Virus (RVFV) is one of the phleboviruses and was first identified in Rift Valley of Africa [73]. Rift Valley fever (RVF) is a zoonotic, vector-borne infectious disease of ruminants and camels transmitted mainly by the *Aedes* and *Culex* mosquito species (**Table 1**). Humans may become infected through contact with the blood or organs of infected animals. This pathogen has led to outbreaks of acute disease, higher abortion rates in cattle, goats, and sheep in Egypt and parts of Africa. The virus is both viscerotropic and neurotropic in these animals. Disease epidemics typically involved thousands to hundreds of thousands of cases of livestock, causing significant economic losses.

2.8.5 Wesselsbron disease

Wesselsbron virus (WSLV) is an RNA virus of the *Flavivirus* genus transmitted by mosquitoes. The disease is widespread across Africa and occurs in cattle and sheep (**Table 1**). In sheep, the disease is clinically similar to RVF and often results in abortions and 20% mortality in pregnant ewes [74].

2.8.6 Myxomatosis (MYX)

The causative agent of MYX is a leporipoxvirus, responsible for myxomatosis, an endemic disease of lagomorphs in parts of South America and the western United States (**Table 1**). Transmission occurs through mechanical biting by arthropods, primarily mosquitoes and fleas. These viruses create dermal, vascularized tumors. Mosquitoes that transmit the virus in Australia include *Culex annulirostris*, *Anopheles annulipes*, and *Aedes* spp.

2.8.7 Dirofilariasis

Two mosquito-transmitted nematodes, *Dirofilaria repens* and *Dirofilaria immitis* (Spirurida: Onchocercidae), hold considerable importance in terms of public health. *Dirofilaria immitis* is responsible for causing severe heartworm disease in dogs and other carnivores, and occasional infections in humans. On the other hand, *D. repens* typically induces a non-pathogenic subcutaneous infection in dogs, yet it stands as the primary causative agent of human dirofilariasis in the Old World (**Table 1**) [75]. Adult *D. immitis* inhabit the right ventricle of the heart muscle and pulmonary arteries of dogs. The worms measure 12–31 cm in length, and when present in large numbers, the infection can also affect the right atrium. *Dirofilaria immitis* causes damage to the endothelium and the integrity of the walls of the pulmonary arteries.

In the heart and pulmonary arteries, fifth-stage larvae develop into sexually mature adults. After mating, around 6–7 months post-infection, females begin releasing microfilariae into the circulation, active embryonic stages measuring about 300 μm long and 7 μm wide. The concentration of microfilariae in the blood varies significantly, from 1000 to 100,000 microfilariae per milliliter. Microfilariae are nocturnal and subperiodic, with peak concentrations in the peripheral blood occurring in the evening. Some dogs never develop microfilaremia, although they support adult *D. immitis*.

Mosquitoes become infected with *D. immitis* when they feed on the blood of an infected dog, ingesting between five and 500 microfilariae in an average 5 mL blood meal. Microfilariae migrate backward into the mosquito's gut within 48 hours after blood intake, where they develop into first-stage larvae. After 8–10 days, larvae progress to the second developmental stage, causing swelling of the Malpighian tubules. After 12–14 days, they become third-stage larvae, which migrate into the mosquito's body cavity [5].

Dirofilaria repens adults live in the subcutaneous tissues of their hosts, surviving for long periods. First-stage larvae (microfilariae) circulate in the bloodstream and are ingested by mosquitoes. These mosquitoes then transmit third-stage larvae (L3) to new hosts during blood meals. While most infections in dogs are asymptomatic, some may show cutaneous symptoms like itching, swelling, skin nodules, and eye inflammation [75].

Vectors of *D. immitis* and *D. repens* vary by geographic area; many mosquito species in several genera are capable of transmission. Grieve et al. (1983) [76] identified 20 species of mosquitoes belonging to the genera *Aedes, Psorophora, Anopheles,* and *Culex*, in which infective *D. immitis* larvae were detected.

2.8.8 Virus chikungunya (CHIK)

Chikungunya virus (CHIKV) is one of the emerging viruses globally. It belongs to the family *Togaviridae* and genus *Alphavirus*, and it is an arthropod-borne virus transmitted by the bite of an infected mosquito, mainly by *Aedes aegypti* and *Aedes albopictus* [77]. Chikungunya virus spreads across tropical areas, causing recurrent outbreaks of chikungunya fever. In recent years, epidemics have affected populations in East and Central Africa, South America, and Southeast Asia (**Table 1**) [78].

CHIKV usually does not cause encephalitic symptoms characteristic of infections with EEE, WEE, and VEE viruses but rather dengue-like arthralgic illness with fever, rash, and severe joint pain.

2.8.9 Sindbis (SIN) virus

The Sindbis virus (SINV) is an alphavirus spread by mosquitoes and found in Eastern Europe, Scandinavia, the former Soviet Union, Asia, Africa, the Middle East, and Australia. Part of the WEE virus complex, it was first isolated from *Culex univittatus* in Egypt in 1952 and causes rash, fever, and muscle and joint pain in humans in Uganda, South Africa, and Australia. The Ockelbo subtype, found in Sweden, Finland, and northern Russia, is transmitted by *Culiseta ochroptera* and likely by *Culex* and *Aedes* mosquitoes, causing similar human illness to SINV [79].

2.8.10 Yellow fever (YF)

Yellow fever is an important zoonotic viral disease that can be fatal for both human and nonhuman primates. It is caused by the yellow fever virus (YFV) (genus *Flavivirus*, family *Flaviviridae*) (**Table 1**) [80]. It occurs in extensive areas of the low equatorial regions of Africa and in South and Central America, either as isolated cases or epidemics. The YFV mainly exists in two epidemiological forms: the enzootic form, maintained in monkey populations by forest mosquitoes in the sylvan cycle and responsible for most isolated cases in humans (jungle yellow fever), and the epidemic form, which spreads rapidly among humans via the domestic form *A. aegypti* in the urban cycle.

2.8.11 Dengue (DEN) virus

The dengue virus (DEN), with four serotypes (dengue 1, 2, 3, and 4), causes dengue fever, dengue hemorrhagic fever (DHF), and dengue shock syndrome (DSS) in humans. Transmitted primarily by *A. aegypti* mosquitoes, DEN is currently found in Southeast Asia, the South Pacific, the Caribbean, Mexico, Central, and South America [81–83]. Past epidemics have occurred in the U.S., Japan, Australia, Greece, and Africa.

Dengue is characterized by fever, rash, severe headache, and muscle and joint pains, earning it the nickname "breakbone fever." Clinical illness develops 5 to 8 days after being bitten by an infected mosquito. Furthermore, DEN has been detected in various animal species, including bats, non-human primates, birds, bovids, dogs, horses, pigs, rodents, marsupials, and other small animals. Apart from bats, acute infections in animals are relatively uncommon (**Table 1**) [84].

2.8.12 ZIKA encephalitis (ZIKA)

The Zika virus (ZIKV) is an important arbovirus belonging to the genus *Flavivirus* of the family *Flaviviridae* (**Table 1**) [84]. This virus was first isolated from sentinel rhesus monkeys in the Zika Forest, Uganda, in 1947, and shortly thereafter from *Aedes africanus* mosquitoes in that forest. The first human cases were documented in Africa in 1952. It has now spread to almost the entire equatorial Africa, to South Asia, including Pakistan, India, Bangladesh, and almost all of Southeast Asia, as well as to many islands in the South Pacific. It has also recently been introduced in Brazil in 2015 and spreading throughout the continental parts of South, Central, and North America, from central Argentina, across the Caribbean islands to the southern United States [84].

2.8.13 West Nile fever (WNF)

West Nile fever (WNF) or West Nile disease (WND) is a viral illness transmitted by mosquitoes, affecting birds, humans, and horses. The virus, known as West Nile virus (WNV), belongs to the *Flavivirus* genus within the *Flaviviridae* family (**Table 1**). WNV is primarily maintained in a cycle between mosquitoes and birds, with humans and horses being incidental hosts. Symptoms in humans and horses can vary from mild febrile illness to severe conditions like meningitis, encephalitis, or even death. The geographical distribution of WNV spans across Europe, Asia, Africa, Australia (where it's known as Kunjin virus), as well as North, Central, and South America. Migratory birds are believed to play a crucial role in spreading the virus, facilitating its reintroduction into regions with sporadic outbreaks. The virus has caused morbidity and mortality in birds, horses, sheep, reptiles, cats, and rodents [85–89]. Over the last two decades, there have been notable increases in human and equine cases.

2.9 Horse flies and deer flies (Tabanidae)

Tabanidae, a diverse family of blood-feeding Diptera, is most abundant in tropical regions but also thrives in moist temperate areas. They are found worldwide except Antarctica and have successfully colonized remote islands like the Galapagos and Melanesian archipelagos, with some species thriving as far north as 60°N latitude [90].

Comprising about 4455 species across 144 genera globally, Tabanidae is among the most diverse families of blood-feeding flies. Notable genera like *Chrysops*, *Hybomitra*, and *Tabanus* include species known for their harmful effects. Deer flies, particularly those in the subfamily Chrysopsinae, such as the genus Chrysops and members of the genus Silvius, are significant pests. Horse flies, represented by Tabanus (107 Nearctic species) and Hybomitra (55 Nearctic species), are also significant pests. In the Old World, Haematopota species, along with *Tabanus* and *Hybomitra*, are notorious pests, while only five *Haematopota* species are found in the Nearctic, with *H. americana* being harmful to mammals.

The term "horse fly" refers to large tabanids, typically 10–30 mm long, known for causing a significant nuisance to livestock and mechanically transmitting various pathogens. These include viruses such as equine infectious anemia, vesicular stomatitis, hog cholera and rinderpest, bacteria (*A. marginale, Bacillus anthracis, Clostridium chauvoei, Pasteurella multocida, F. tularensis, Brucella spp., L. monocytogenes, Erysiphelothrix rhusiopathiae*), protozoa (*Besnoitia besnoiti, Trypanosoma evansi, Trypanosoma equiperdum, Trypanosoma congolense, Trypanosoma brucei brucei, Trypanosoma b. gambiense (rhodesiense)*), and nematodes (*Loa loa, D. repens, D. roemeri, Elaeophora schneideri, Onchocerca gibsoni*) (**Table 1**). *Trypanosoma evansi*, transmitted by tabanids, causes surra, a serious disease affecting livestock. Unlike transmission by tsetse flies, transmission of *T. evansi* by tabanids is mechanical, and the pathogen can be transmitted through contaminated blood. Surra affects various mammals in different regions worldwide, and untreated infections are often fatal. Another trypanosome, *T. theileri*, often infects cattle and wild domestic animals without causing serious illness. Even a moderate number of flies feeding on livestock can lead to significant production losses.

Smaller tabanid species known as clegs typically measure 6–11 mm in length. Unlike horse flies, they often attack humans. The most important diseases transmitted by tabanids are loiasis and tularemia.

Tabanids, due to their painful and persistent biting habits, pose a significant challenge to livestock, especially cattle and horses, and are extremely irritating to many wild animal species. Intense tabanid attacks can directly reduce weight gain in beef cattle, milk yield, and feed efficiency and cause skin damage from bites [90].

2.10 Muscid flies (Muscidae)

The Muscidae family encompasses approximately 5000 species in 200 genera [91]. Important muscids are found in two subfamilies: Muscinae and Fanniinae. Species from the Muscidae family include significant hematophagous parasites, disease vector species, and those that irritate humans and domestic animals. Flies and their relatives can be grouped according to their habitat affinities. There are filth flies, such as the housefly, whose adult individuals and larvae inhabit various filthy organic substrates, including household waste, livestock manure, and bedding soiled with animal excrement. A subset of filth flies are those that develop exclusively in dung, such as horn flies, whose larvae are found solely in the feces of livestock [91].

Adult individuals and larvae of some important Muscidae flies can be preliminarily identified based on their external characteristics and behaviors, habitats, and geographic locations.

Muscid flies are significant veterinary pests that impact the health and comfort of both domestic and wild animals. They target domestic hosts like cattle, sheep, goats, horses, dogs, pigs, and poultry, while in North America, they also affect wild animals [91]. These flies cause discomfort, skin injuries, hinder growth, and transmit pathogenic viruses, bacteria, helminths, and cestodes. Their feeding and biting can lead to secondary infections and crust formation on animals' ears, legs, back, and other areas. Non-biting flies can also impede wound healing caused by arthropod bites and other factors. Muscidae fly larvae are involved in secondary myiasis in mammals and primary myiasis in birds.

The Housefly (*Musca domestica*) is the most numerous insect around livestock, poultry, or pets. Therefore, it is important to note that houseflies can be significant mechanical carriers of microbial pathogens. Adult individuals feed on feces and manure, contaminating the environment with flies. These habits contribute to microbial contamination of eggs and milk at production points.

Houseflies are also developmental hosts for *Draschia megastoma, Habronema majus*, and *Habronema muscae* spirurid nematodes that cause gastric and cutaneous forms of habronemiasis in horses (**Table 1**). Females go to wound sites to feed and lay eggs. Later, larvae feed on wound secretions and slow down healing.

2.11 Tsetse flies (Glossinidae)

Tsetse flies are obligatory hematophagous insects of medical and veterinary significance because they transmit trypanosomes that cause African sleeping sickness in humans and African animal trypanosomosis (nagana) disease in domestic and wild animals (**Table 1**). Tsetse flies are now found across more than 10 million square kilometers in tropical and subtropical regions of sub-Saharan Africa [5, 92].

Most wild hosts in Africa are immune to these parasites or have inconspicuous or mild infections [93]. However, more than 30 species of wild animals indigenous to Africa carry trypanosomes (reservoirs) that are pathogenic when transmitted to domestic animals.

2.11.1 Nagana

Trypanosoma brucei spp. causes African sleeping sickness in humans (human African trypanosomiasis) and nagana disease in livestock (Animal African trypanosomiasis). *Trypanosoma brucei gambiense* and *T. b. rhodesiense* subspecies infect both humans and animals, while *T. b. brucei* only infects animals [94].

Nagana significantly impacts commercial domestic animal production across approximately one-third of Africa (**Table 1**). Between 40 and 60 million cattle and millions of sheep, goats, horses, donkeys, pigs, and camels are at risk of infection. Unlike African sleeping sickness, which is limited to regions with tsetse fly vectors, nagana occurs wherever tsetse flies are present. In some areas, infection can also spread through mechanical transmission by other blood-sucking insects.

The course of the disease in cattle and pigs is relatively mild, while in sheep and goats it is moderate and in horses, donkeys, and dogs it is quite severe [95]. Disease symptoms include fever, lethargy, exhaustion, decreased milk production, hair loss, discharge from the eyes, edema, anemia, and paralysis [96]. As the disease progresses, animals become weaker and eventually unable to work. Chronic disease involving anemia and weakness is common.

2.12 Myiasis (Muscoidea, Oestroidea)

Myiasis is the infestation of host tissues by larval stages of dipterous flies, known as maggots or grubs, which feed on the host's necrotic or living tissue. Hosts typically include mammals, birds, amphibians, or reptiles. The economically significant agents of veterinary myiasis belong to the calyptrate Diptera in the superfamily Oestroidea. This superfamily includes three main families of myiasis-causing flies: Oestridae, Calliphoridae, and Sarcophagidae.

Oestrinae contains the genus *Oestrus*, along with *Rhinoestrus*, *Cephenemyia*, and *Cephalopina*. Gasterophilinae includes the significant genus *Gasterophilus*. Hypodermatinae contains *Hypoderma* and *Przhevalskiana*. Cuterebrinae includes *Cuterebra* and Dermatobia. These are obligate parasites with a high level of host specificity, causing dermal, subdermal, cutaneous, nasopharyngeal, ocular, intestinal/enteric, or urogenital myiasis. Three types of facultative myiasis are recognized: primary myiasis involves species capable of initiating myiasis; secondary myiasis involves species that continue myiasis after being initiated by primary species; and tertiary myiasis involves species that join primary and secondary species shortly before the host's death [96].

Many or even most of these facultative flies usually feed on dead, decomposing tissue rather than invading healthy tissue (e.g., screw-worms), but they can transition from dead to live tissue and vice versa easily (e.g., *Cochliomyia macellaria*, *Wohlfahrtia nuba*). In a way, they are opportunistic parasites that can infest a sick or injured host and complete their larval development after the host's death. Adult flies are attracted to open wounds or chronic surface wounds with purulent exudates.

In obligatory myiasis, fly larvae are always parasitic and require a live host for their development. Examples include primary bots and warbles. This category includes species that cause temporary myiasis, involving occasional contact between fly larvae and their host, such as larvae in nests and larvae on the ground. In this form of myiasis, the larvae do not remain in constant contact with their host. When flies causing obligatory myiasis occasionally parasitize atypical hosts, it is termed accidental myiasis.

Gastrointestinal myiasis involves the presence of fly larvae in the host's digestive tract, which can occur accidentally (such as through the ingestion of eggs or larvae of false stable flies in uncooked fruits) or obligatorily, as observed in the development of horse bot larvae. Urogenital myiasis occurs when fly larvae invade the urethra and/or genitalia. Ophthalmic myiasis, predominantly caused by sheep nose flies (*Oestrus ovis*), involves the invasion of eye tissues by larvae, although other fly species from various subfamilies can also be implicated.

2.13 Louse flies, Keds, and bat flies

Members of the families Hippoboscidae, Streblidae, and Nycteribiidae are obligatory hematophagous ectoparasites, forming the superfamily Hippoboscoidea with Glossinidae. While Hippoboscidae are known by various names like louse flies and tick flies, mostly parasitizing birds with some on bats, Streblidae and Nycteribiidae (**Figure 11**), exclusively parasitize bats. Despite their close association with bats, these insects rarely bother or bite humans, even in settings where bats infest attics or buildings [5].

Young birds and mammals are more heavily infested with hippoboscids than older animals. These parasites can worsen the condition of hibernating hosts, and their presence causes discomfort and irritation due to biting and crawling [97, 98]. The diversity of Hippoboscoidea mainly includes ectoparasites of bats. Despite limited studies on disease transmission, these ectoparasites exhibit potential as effective vectors due to their blood-feeding habits and interactions within bat colonies. Arboviruses and *Bartonella* spp. have been isolated from nycteribiids in Spain and Africa [99]. Ecological studies of *Bartonella* infections in bats associate parasite abundance with infections. A rhabdovirus discovered in Spanish bats was also found in both bats and nycteribiids, indicating infection in both hosts. Streblids have also been linked to potential bat pathogens, including *Bartonella* spp. Furthermore, DNA of filarial nematodes, *Litomosoides* spp., has been detected in *Trichobius intermedius*, suggesting bats as definitive hosts for several *Litomosoides* spp., with mites or bat flies suspected as vectors.

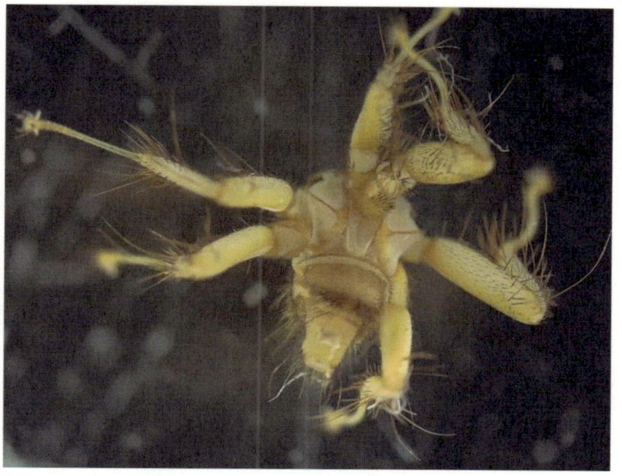

Figure 11.
Nycteribiidae flies [6].

Many nycteribiid species are presumed vectors of *Polychromophilus* spp., haemosporidian parasites of bats in the Old World, as well as *Trypanosoma vespertilionis* [100].

Sheep keds have been shown in experiments to transmit BTV. Although *C. burnetii* has been detected in various bloodsucking insects, sheep keds removed from infected sheep flocks have not been observed to transmit this pathogen, although this does not definitively prove they cannot. Sheep keds were also found incapable of transmitting *Anaplasma ovis* between infected and uninfected sheep. Furthermore, the sheep ked (*Lipoptena fortisetosa*) is associated with potential endosymbionts *Coxiella* spp. and *Theileria* spp., but there is no evidence confirming their transmission to their hosts [101].

3. Conclusion

It has been concluded that arthropods cause significant economic losses worldwide and negatively impact livestock hosts in various ways, parasitizing a wide range of vertebrate hosts and transmitting a diverse array of pathogenic agents. Effective control of arthropod-borne diseases requires a better understanding of the interactions among hosts, vectors, and pathogens. Concurrently, while insecticides and acaricides are still widely used, they present serious ecological problems and contribute to the development of resistance in arthropods. More appropriate control and sustainable use of antiparasitics can be achieved by focusing on threshold-based disease management and understanding that the primary causes of many animal health issues may be factors affecting the animals' susceptibility rather than the parasites themselves. Despite significant progress and encouraging results, ongoing efforts are needed to deepen our understanding of host-arthropod-pathogen interactions.

Author details

Jasmin Omeragić[1], Naida Kapo[1*], Vedad Škapur[2], Šejla Goletić[1], Adis Softić[1], Ermin Šaljić[1] and Teufik Goletić[1]

1 Veterinary Faculty, University of Sarajevo, Bosnia and Herzegovina

2 Faculty of Agriculture and Food Science, University of Sarajevo, Bosnia and Herzegovina

*Address all correspondence to: naida.kapo@vfs.unsa.ba

IntechOpen

© 2024 The Author(s). Licensee IntechOpen. This chapter is distributed under the terms of the Creative Commons Attribution License (http://creativecommons.org/licenses/by/4.0), which permits unrestricted use, distribution, and reproduction in any medium, provided the original work is properly cited.

References

[1] Santos JC, de Almeida WR, Fernandes GW. Arthropods: Why it is so crucial to know their biodiversity? In: Santos JC, Fernandes GW, editors. Measuring Arthropod Biodiversity. Cham: Springer; 2021

[2] Ødegaard F. How many species of arthropods? Erwin's estimate revised. Biological Journal of the Linnean Society. 2000;**71**:583-597. DOI: 10.1111/j.1095-8312.2000.tb01279.x

[3] Gillott C. Entomology. Springer Science & Business Media. New York: Plenum Press; 2005

[4] Mathison BA, Pritt BS. Laboratory identification of arthropod ectoparasites. Clinical Microbiology Reviews. 2014;**27**:48-67. DOI: 10.1128/cmr.00008-13

[5] Mullen GR, Durden LA. Medical and Veterinary Entomology. Elsevier, Academic Press; 2019

[6] Omeragic J, Jažić A, Zuko A. Handbook of Veterinary Parasitology. Sarajevo: University of Sarajevo-Veterinary Faculty; 2018

[7] Estrada-Pena A, Mangold AJ, Nava S, Venzal JM, Labruna M, Guglielmone AA. A review of the systematics of the tick family Argasidae (Ixodida). Acarologia. 2010;**50**:317-333. DOI: 10.1051/acarologia/20101975

[8] Krantz GW, Walter DE. A Manual of Acarology. 3rd ed. Lubbock, Texas: Texas Tech University Press; 2009

[9] Guglielmone AA, Robbins RG, Apanaskevich DA, Petney TN, Estrada-Peña A, Horak IG, et al. The Argasidae, Ixodidae and Nuttalliellidae (Acari: Ixodida) of the world: A list of valid species names. Zootaxa. 2010;**2528**:1. DOI: 10.11646/zootaxa.2528.1.1

[10] Bartíková P, Holíková V, Kazimírová M, Štibrániová I. Tick-borne viruses. Acta Virologica. 2017;**61**:413-427

[11] Snelson JT. Animal ectoparasites and disease vector causing major reduction in world food supplies. FAO Plant Protection Bulleton. 1975;**13**:103-114

[12] Oliver JH. Biology and systematics of ticks (Acari: Ixodida). Annual Review of Ecology and Systematics. 1989;**20**(1):397-430. DOI: 10.1146/annurev.es.20.110189.002145

[13] Paucar-Quishpe V, Pérez-Otáñez X, Rodríguez-Hidalgo R, Cepeda-Bastidas D, Pérez-Escalante C, Grijalva-Olmedo J, et al. An economic evaluation of cattle tick acaricide-resistances and the financial losses in subtropical dairy farms of Ecuador: A farm system approach. PLoS One. 2023;**18**(6):e0287104. DOI: 10.1371/journal.pone.0287104

[14] Clow KM, Ogden NH, Lindsay LR, Michel P, Pearl DL, Jardine CM. Distribution of ticks and the risk of Lyme disease and other tick-borne pathogens of public health significance in Ontario, Canada. Vector-Borne and Zoonotic Diseases. 2016;**16**(4):215-222. DOI: 10.1089/vbz.2015.1890

[15] Kazimírová M, Thangamani S, Bartíková P, Hermance M, Holíková V, Štibrániová I, et al. Tick-borne viruses and biological processes at the tick-host-virus interface. Frontiers in Cellular and Infection Microbiology. 2017;**7**:339. DOI: 10.3389/fcimb.2017.00339

[16] Dantas-Torres F, Chomel BB, Otranto D. Ticks and tick-borne diseases: A one health perspective. Trends in Parasitology. 2012;**28**(10):437-446. DOI: 10.1016/j.pt.2012.07.003

[17] Krasteva S, Jara M, Frias-De-Diego A, Machado G. Nairobi sheep disease virus: A historical and epidemiological perspective. Frontiers in Veterinary Science. 2020;**7**:419. DOI: 10.3389/fvets.2020.00419

[18] Mertens M, Schmidt K, Ozkul A, Groschup MH. The impact of Crimean-Congo hemorrhagic fever virus on public health. Antiviral Research. 2013;**98**(2):248-260. DOI: 10.1016/j.antiviral.2013.02.007

[19] Stanek G, Wormser GP, Gray J, Strle F. Lyme borreliosis. The Lancet. 2012;**379**(9814):461-473. DOI: 10.1016/s0140-6736(11)60103-7

[20] Gyuranecz M, Rigó K, Dán Á, Földvári G, Makrai L, Dénes B, et al. Investigation of the ecology of *Francisella tularensis* during an inter-epizootic period. Vector-Borne and Zoonotic Diseases. 2011;**11**(8):1031-1035. DOI: 10.1089/vbz.2010.0091

[21] Dumler JS, Barbet AF, Bekker CP, Dasch GA, Palmer GH, Ray SC, et al. Reorganization of genera in the families Rickettsiaceae and Anaplasmataceae in the order Rickettsiales: Unification of some species of *Ehrlichia* with *Anaplasma*, *Cowdria* with *Ehrlichia* and *Ehrlichia* with *Neorickettsia*, descriptions of six new species combinations and designation of *Ehrlichia equi* and "HGE agent" as subjective synonyms of *Ehrlichia phagocytophila*. International Journal of Systematic and Evolutionary Microbiology. 2001;**51**(6):2145-2165. DOI: 10.1099/00207713-51-6-2145

[22] Atif FA. *Anaplasma marginale* and *Anaplasma phagocytophilum*: Rickettsiales pathogens of veterinary and public health significance. Parasitology Research. 2015;**114**(11):3941-3957. DOI: 10.1007/s00436-015-4698-2

[23] Allsopp BA. Natural history of *Ehrlichia ruminantium*. Veterinary Parasitology. 2010;**167**(2-4):123-135. DOI: 10.1016/j.vetpar.2009.09.014

[24] Brites-Neto J, Duarte KMR, Martins TF. Tick-borne infections in human and animal population worldwide. Veterinary World. 2015;**8**(3):301-315. DOI: 10.14202/vetworld.2015.301-315

[25] Bano S, Lodh C. Epidemiological studies on canine babesiosis. Indian Journal of Canine Practice. 2019;**11**(1):090. DOI: 10.29005/ijcp.2019.11.1.090-093

[26] Zhang ZQ, editor. Animal biodiversity: An outline of higher-level classification and survey of taxonomic richness. Zootaxa. 2011;**3148**:1-237

[27] Fields PG. The control of stored-product insects and mites with extreme temperatures. Journal of Stored Products Research. 1992;**28**:89-118. DOI: 10.1016/0022-474X(92)90018-L

[28] Sparagano O, Pavlićević A, Murano T, Camarda A, Sahibi H, Kilpinen O, et al. Prevalence and key figures for the poultry red mite Dermanyssus gallinae infections in poultry farm systems. Experimental & Applied Acarology. 2009;**48**(1-2):3-10. DOI: 10.1007/s10493-008-9233-z

[29] Sweatman GK. Parasitic mites of nondomesticated animals in New Zealand. The New Zealand Entomologist. 1962;**3**(1):15-23

[30] Wharton GW, Fuller HS. A Manual of the Chiggers: The Biology, Classification, Distribution and

Importance to Man of the Larvae of the Family Trombiculidae (Acarina). The University of Michigan, Entomology Society of Washington; 1952. p. 185

[31] Jiang J, Richards AL. Scrub typhus: No longer restricted to the Tsutsugamushi triangle. Tropical Medicine and Infectious Disease. 2018;**3**(1):11

[32] Curtis CF. Current trends in the treatment of Sarcoptes, Cheyletiella and Otodectes mite infestations in dogs and cats. Veterinary Dermatology. 2004;**15**(2):108-114

[33] Muller GH, Kirk RW. Dermatología en pequeños animales. 4th ed. Buenos Aires, Argentina: Interamericana; 1991

[34] Choi WP, Lee SI, Lee KW. Etiological and epidemiological features of canine dermatitis. Korean Journal of Veterinary Research. 2000;**40**(1):94-100

[35] Fain A, Bochkov AV. New species of mites parasitic on the skin of birds (Acari Epidermoptidae and Dermationidae). Bulletin of the Royal Belgium Entomology. 2003;**139**:121-149

[36] Lacey N, Raghallaigh S, Powell F. *Demodex* mites–commensals, parasites or mutualistic organisms? Dermatology. 2011;**222**:128-130

[37] Jacob S, VanDaele MA, Brown JN. Treatment of *Demodex*-associated inflammatory skin conditions: A systematic review. Dermatologic Therapy. 2019;**32**(6):e13103

[38] Sastre N, Francino O, Curti JN, Armenta TC, Fraser DL, Kelly RM, et al. Detection, prevalence and phylogenetic relationships of *Demodex* spp. and further skin Prostigmata mites (Acari, Arachnida) in wild and domestic mammals. PLoS One. 2016;**11**(11):e0165765. DOI: 10.1371/journal.pone.0165765

[39] Foley J, Serieys LEK, Stephenson N, Riley S, Foley C, Jennings M, et al. A synthetic review of notoedres species mites and mange. Parasitology. 2016;**143**(14):1847-1861

[40] Bochkov AV, Saveljev AP. Mites of the genus Schizocarpus Trouessart, 1896 (Acariformes: Chirodiscidae) from the north American beavers (*Castor canadensis*) in Russia. Parazitologiya (St. Petersburg). 2014;**48**:430-436

[41] Sweatman GK. On the life history and validity of the species in psoroptes, a genus of mange mites. Canadian Journal of Zoology. 1958;**36**:905-929

[42] Kouchakji GA, Loos-Frank B. The validity and morphology of lung mites of the genus Pneumocoptes (Acari: Astigmata). Zeitschrift für Parasitenkunde. 1984;**70**:673-683

[43] Fain A. Observations sur les Rodhainyssinae acariens parasites des voies respiratoires des chauves-souris (Gastronyssidae: Sarcoptiformes). Acta Zoologica et Pathologica Antverpiensia. 1967;**44**:3-35

[44] Arther RG. Mites and lice: Biology and control. Veterinary Clinics: Small Animal Practice. 2009;**39**(6):1159-1171

[45] Ramakrishnan MA, Ashokkumar D. Swinepox virus. In: Malik Y, Singh R, Yadav M, editors. Recent Advances in Animal Virology. Singapore: Springer; 2019. DOI: 10.1007/978-981-13-9073-9_9

[46] Acosta DB, Ruiz M, Sanchez JP. First molecular detection of *mycoplasma suis* in the pig louse *Haematopinus suis* (Phthiraptera: Anoplura)

from Argentina. Acta Tropica. 2019;**194**:165-168

[47] Cabello RR, Ruiz AC, Feregrino RR, Romero LC, Feregrino RR, Zavala JT. *Dipylidium caninum* infection. Case Reports. 2011;**2011**:bcr0720114510

[48] Zhu Q, Hastriter MW, Whiting MF, Dittmar K. Fleas(Siphonaptera) are cretaceous, and evolved with Theria. Molecular Phylogenetics and Evolution. 2015;**90**:129-e139

[49] Beck W, Boch K, Mackensen H, Wiegand B, Pfister K. Qualitative and quantitative observations on the flea population dynamics of dogs and cats in several areas of Germany. Veterinary Parasitology. 2006;**137**:130-136

[50] Marchiondo AA, Holdsworth PA, Green P, Blagburn BL, Jacobs DE. World Association for the Advancement of Veterinary Parasitology (W.A.A.V.P.) guidelines for evaluating the efficacy of parasiticides for the treatment, prevention and control of flea and tick infestation on dogs and cats. Veterinary Parasitology. 2007;**145**:332-344

[51] Linardi PM, Santos JLC. *Ctenocephalides felis felis* vs. *Ctenocephalides canis* (Siphonaptera: Pulicidae): Some issues in correctly identify these species. Revista Brasileira de Parasitologia Veterinária. 2012;**21**(4):345-354. DOI: 10.1590/s1984-29612012000400002

[52] Tripet F, Richner H. The coevolutionary potential of a 'generalist' parasite, the hen flea *Ceratophyllus gallinae*. Parasitology. 1997;**115**:419-427

[53] Hustedt J, Prasetyo DB, Fiorenzano JM, et al. Phlebotomine sand flies (Diptera: Psychodidae) and sand fly-borne pathogens in the greater Mekong subregion: A systematic review. Parasites and Vectors. 2022;**15**:355. DOI: 10.1186/s13071-022-05464-8

[54] Depaquit N, Léger. Les phlébotomes (Diptera: Psychodidae: Phlebotominae). In: Duvallet G, Fontenille D, Roert V, editors. Entomologie médicale et vétérinaire. Marseille: IRD Éditions; 2017. pp. 295-320

[55] Maia C. Sand fly-borne diseases in Europe: Epidemiological overview and potential triggers for their emergence and re-emergence. Journal of Comparative Pathology. 2024;**209**:6-12

[56] Serrano C, García E, León V, Rosiles M. Enfermedad de Carrión. Revista Mexicana de Patología Clínica y Medicina de Laboratorio. 2014;**61**:246-252

[57] Christodoulou V, Antoniou M, Ntais P, Messaritakis I, Ivovic V, Dedet J-P, et al. Re-emergence of visceral and cutaneous Leishmaniasis in the Greek Island of Crete. Vector Borne and Zoonotic Diseases. 2012;**12**:214-222

[58] Koliou MG, Antoniou Y, Antoniou M, Christodoulou V, Mazeris A, Soteriades ES. A cluster of four cases of cutaneous leishmaniasis by *Leishmania donovani* in Cyprus: A case series. Journal of Medical Case Reports. 2014;**8**:354

[59] Maclachlan NJ, Zientara S, Savini G, Daniels PW. Epizootic haemorrhagic disease. Revue Scientifique et Technique. 2015;**34**:341-351

[60] Hassine TB, Amdouni J, Monaco F, Savini G, Sghaier S, Selimen IB, et al. Emerging vector-borne diseases in dromedaries in Tunisia: West Nile, bluetongue, epizootic haemorrhagic disease and Rift Valley fever. The Onderstepoort Journal of Veterinary Research. 2017;**84**:e1-e3

[61] Kamomae Y, Kamomae M, Ohta Y, Nabe M, Kagawa Y, Ogura Y, et al. Epizootic hemorrhagic disease virus serotype 6 infection in cattle, Japan, 2015. Emerging Infectious Diseases. 2018;**24**:902-905

[62] Golender N, Khinich Y, Gorohov A, Abramovitz I, Bumbarov V. Epizootic hemorrhagic disease virus serotype 6 outbreak in Israeli cattle in 2015. Journal of Veterinary Diagnostic Investigation. 2017;**29**:885-888

[63] Larska M, Lechowski L, Grochowska M, Zmudzinski JF. Detection of the Schmallenberg virus in nulliparous *Culicoides obsoletus/scoticus* complex and *C. punctatus*: The possibility of transovarial virus transmission in the midge population and of a new vector. Veterinary Microbiology. 2013;**166**:467-473

[64] Saminathan M, Singh KP, Khorajiya JH, Dinesh M, Vineetha S, Madhulina Maity AT, et al. An updated review on bluetongue virus: Epidemiology, pathobiology, and advances in diagnosis and control with special reference to India. Veterinary Quarterly. 2020;**40**(1):258-321. DOI: 10.1080/01652176.2020.1831708

[65] MacLachlan NJ, Drew CP, Darpel KE, Worwa G. The pathology and pathogenesis of bluetongue. Journal of Comparative Pathology. 2009;**141**:1-16

[66] Adler PH, Kúdelová T, Kúdela M, Seitz G, Ignjatovic-Cupina A. Cryptic biodiversity and the origins of pest status revealed in the macrogenome of *Simulium colombaschense* (Diptera: Simuliidae), history's most destructive black fly. PLoS One. 2016;**11**(1):e0147673

[67] Adler PH, Cheke RA, Post RJ. Evolution, epidemiology, and population genetics of black flies (Diptera: Simuliidae). Infection, Genetics and Evolution. 2010;**10**:846-865

[68] Adler PH. Black flies, the Simuliidae. In: Marquardt WC, editor. Biology of Disease Vectors. London, UK: Elsevier Academic Press; 2004. pp. 127-141

[69] Woolhouse MEJ, Webster JP, Domingo E, Charlesworth B, Levin BR. Biological and biomedical implications of the co-evolution of pathogens and their hosts. Nature Genetics. 2002;**32**:569-577

[70] Corrin T, Ackford R, Mascarenhas M, Greig J, Waddell LA. Eastern equine encephalitis virus: A scoping review of the global evidence. Vector-Borne and Zoonotic Diseases. 2021;**21**(5):305-320. DOI: 10.1089/vbz.2020.2671

[71] Forrester NL, Kenney JL, Deardorff E, Wang E, Weaver SC. Western equine encephalitis submergence: Lack of evidence for a decline in virus virulence. Virology. 2008;**380**(2):170-172

[72] Hsieh JT, St. John AL. Japanese encephalitis virus and its mechanisms of neuroinvasion. PLoS Pathogens. 2020;**16**(4):e1008260. DOI: 10.1371/journal.ppat.1008260

[73] Daubney R, Hudson JR. Enzootic hepatitis or Rift Valley fever. An undescribed virus disease of sheep cattle and man from East Africa. The Journal of Pathology and Bacteriology. 1931;**34**:545-579

[74] Kayiwa JT, Mayanja MN, Nakayiki TM, Senfuka F, Mugga J, Koehler JW, et al. Phylogenetic analysis of Wesselsbron virus isolated from field-captured mosquitoes during a Rift Valley fever outbreak in Kabale District, Uganda-2016. The American Journal of Tropical Medicine and Hygiene.

2022;**108**(1):161-164. DOI: 10.4269/ajtmh.22-0481

[75] Pampiglione S, Rivasi F. Human dirofilariasis due to *Dirofilaria* (Nochtiella) *repens*: An update of world literature from 1995 to 2000. Parassitologia. 2000;**42**:231-254

[76] Grieve RB, Lok JB, Glickman LT. Epidemiology of canine heartworm infection. Epidemiologic Reviews. 1983;**5**:220-246

[77] Manzoor KN, Javed F, Ejaz M, et al. The global emergence of chikungunya infection: An integrated view. Reviews in Medical Virology. 2022;**32**(3):e2287. DOI: 10.1002/rmv.2287

[78] Bartholomeeusen K, Daniel M, LaBeaud DA, et al. Chikungunya fever. Nature Reviews. Disease Primers. 2023;**9**:17. DOI: 10.1038/s41572-023-00429-2

[79] Uusitalo R, Siljander M, Culverwell CL, Hendrickx G, Lindén A, Dub T, et al. Predicting spatial patterns of Sindbis virus (SINV) infection risk in Finland using vector, host and environmental data. International Journal of Environmental Research and Public Health. 2021;**18**:7064. DOI: 10.3390/ijerph18137064

[80] Lindenbach BD, Murray CL, Thiel HJ, Rice CM. Flaviviridae. In: Knipe DM, Howley PM, editors. Fields Virology. Philadelphia: Lippincot William & Wilkins; 2013

[81] PFdC V, JAS Q. Yellow fever. In: Mehlhorn H, Heukelbach J, editors. Infectious Tropical Diseases and One Health in Latin America. Parasitology Research Monographs, Vol 16. Cham: Springer; 2022. DOI: 10.1007/978-3-030-99712-0_1

[82] Guzman MG, Harris E. Dengue. The Lancet. 2015;**385**(9966):453-465

[83] Gwee SXW, St John AL, Gray GC, Pang J. Animals as potential reservoirs for dengue transmission: A systematic review. One Health (Amsterdam, Netherlands). 2021;**12**:100216. DOI: 10.1016/j.onehlt.2021.100216

[84] Sharma V, Sharma M, Dhull D, Sharma Y, Kaushik S, Kaushik S. Zika virus: An emerging challenge to public health worldwide. Canadian Journal of Microbiology. 2019;**66**(2):87-98. DOI: 10.1139/cjm-2019-0331

[85] Stockman J, Hawkins MG, Burns RE, Fang Y, Brault AC, Lowenstine LJ. West Nile virus infection in a green-winged macaw (*Ara chloropterus*). Avian Diseases. 2010;**54**:164-169

[86] Cardinale E, Bernard C, Lecollinet S, Rakotoharinome VM, Ravaomanana J, Roger M, et al. West Nile virus infection in horses, Indian ocean. Comparative Immunology, Microbiology and Infectious Diseases. 2017;**53**:45-49

[87] Rimoldi G, Mete A, Adaska J, Anderson M, Symmes K, Diab S. West Nile virus infection in sheep. Veterinary Pathology. 2017;**54**:155-158

[88] Dahlin CR, Hughes DF, Meshaka WE, Coleman C, Henning JD. Wild snakes harbor West Nile virus. One Health. 2016;**2**:136-138

[89] Marschang RE. Viruses infecting reptiles. Viruses. 2011;**3**:2087-2126

[90] Mullens BA. Horse flies and deer flies (Tabanidae). In: Medical and Veterinary Entomology. Academic Press, Elsevier; 2019. pp. 327-343. DOI: 10.1016/b978-0-12-814043-7.00016-9

[91] Moon RD. Muscid flies (Muscidae). In: Medical and Veterinary

Entomology. Academic Press, Elsevier; 2019. pp. 345-368. DOI: 10.1016/b978-0-12-814043-7.00017-0

[92] Elsen P, Amoudi MA, Leclercq M. First record of *Glossina fuscipes fuscipes* Newstead, 1910 and *Glossina morsitans submorsitans* Newstead, 1910 in southwestern Saudi Arabia. Annales de Societé de Belge Médecin Tropicale. 1990;**70**:281-287

[93] Ford J. The Role of the Trypanosomiases in African Ecologyea Study of the Tsetse Fly Problem. Oxford: Clarendon Press; 1971

[94] McKelvey JJ Jr. Man against Tsetse: Struggle for Africa. Ithaca: Cornell University Press; 1973. 306 p

[95] Taylor K, Authié EML. Pathogenesis of animal trypanosomiasis. In: Maudlin I, Holmes PH, Miles MA, editors. The Trypanosomiases. CABI: Wallingford; 2004. pp. 331-353

[96] Kettle DS. Medical and Veterinary Entomology. 2nd ed. Cambridge: C.A.B. International, UK at the University Press; 1995. 725 p

[97] Davis AK. Can a blood-feeding ectoparasitic fly affect songbird migration? Examining body condition and fat reserves of five bird species in relation to hippoboscid fly parasitism. Ecological Parasitology and Immunology. 2015;**4**:235907. DOI: 10.4303/epi/235907

[98] Linhares AX, Komeno CA. *Trichobius joblingi*, *Aspidoptera falcata*, and *Megistopoda proxima* (Diptera: Streblidae) parasitic on *Carolla perspicilllata* and *Sturnira lillum* (Chiroptera: Phyllostomidae) in southeastern Brazil: Sex ratios, seasonality, host site preference, and effect of parasitism on the host. The Journal of Parasitology. 2000;**86**:167-170

[99] Aznar-Lopez C, Vazquez-Moron S, Marston DA, Juste J, Ibanez C, Berciano JM, et al. Detection of Rhabdovirus viral RNA in oropharyngeal swabs and ectoparasites of Spanish bats. The Journal of General Virology. 2013;**94**:69-75

[100] Hoare CA. The Trypanosomes of Mammals. Oxford: Blackwell Scientific Publications; 1972

[101] Lee SH, Kim KT, Kwon OD, Ock Y, Kim T, Choi D, et al. Novel detection of *Coxiella* spp., *Theileria luwenshuni*, and *T. ovis* endosymbionts in deer Keds (*Lipoptena fortisetosa*). PLoS One. 2016;**11**(5):e0156727. DOI: 10.1371/journal.pone.0156727

Chapter 4

Rift Valley Fever Virus

Binu T. Velayudhan and Shaun van den Hurk

Abstract

Rift Valley fever virus (RVFV) is a negative-sense, single-stranded RNA virus in the genus Phlebovirus of the family Phenuviridae. It is an arbovirus transmitted mainly by mosquitoes. RVFV is an emerging zoonotic disease where humans can get infected *via* exposure of mucosa or broken skin to infected animals or through mosquito transmission. The disease was first detected in sheep in the Rift Valley region in Kenya in 1930, and since then, several outbreaks have been reported in northern and sub-Saharan Africa and Middle Eastern countries. North America is considered free of RVF, but the mosquito vectors involved in the transmission of RVF are present in many regions of the American and European continents. The virus causes disease in livestock characterized by hemorrhagic fever. The severity of the disease varies among different species, with sheep experiencing the most severe infection. Young as well as pregnant animals may also be severely affected by RVFV. For laboratory diagnosis, reverse transcription-quantitative polymerase chain reaction (RT-qPCR) is the most commonly used test. Other assays, including serological assays and nucleic acid-based point-of-care tests, are also available for RVF diagnosis. There is no specific treatment for RVFV infection. Control and preventive measures should include vaccination, vector control, and proper hygiene.

Keywords: Rift Valley fever virus, vector-borne, hemorrhagic fever, zoonosis, livestock disease

1. Introduction

Rift Valley fever (RVF) is an important mosquito-borne zoonotic disease. The disease is caused by the Rift Valley fever virus (RVFV) and primarily affects livestock. However, a large number of cases have been reported in humans, with these cases ranging in severity [1, 2]. RVF is typically classified as a hemorrhagic fever disease, although high abortion rates may be a distinct identifier in outbreaks in naïve domestic ruminant flocks and herds. The virus and disease are named after the Rift Valley region in Kenya, where it was first diagnosed in 1930 [1]. Since then, RVFV has been observed in most parts of the African continent, with sporadic and cyclic outbreaks in numerous countries [1–3]. Of great concern is the fact that more recently, there has been increased evidence of spread beyond the African continent, with cases in the Middle East and Arabian Peninsula, and even the transport of suspect cases to Europe [4–9].

2. Etiology and epidemiology

Rift Valley fever virus is a *Phlebovirus* in the *Phenuviridae* family, which is in the *Bunyavirales* order [10]. It is an enveloped negative-sense RNA virus with a spherical or pleomorphic structure and is approximately 100 nm in diameter [11]. The viral genome consists of three main components, the S (small), M (medium), and L (large) segments, which are encapsulated by the ribonucleoprotein (RNP) complex, which includes the N (nucleocapsid) protein [10–12]. Among other translation sites, the M segment encodes a glycoprotein precursor (GPC), which is cleaved into the structural glycoproteins Gn and Gc [1, 12, 13]. These glycoproteins have essential functions in virus entry and fusion, thereby facilitating host-cell entry. Thereafter, as a negative-sense virus, the L segment encodes viral RNA-dependent RNA polymerase (RdRp), which is essential for viral replication [14]. The small segment produces the N and NS (nonstructural) proteins, and these are essential for viral replication as well as being recognized as the primary virulence factors for infection [14–16].

Rift Valley fever is a mosquito-borne infection, and therefore, transmission is largely dependent on mosquito vectors and the prevailing conditions that may affect their populations and distribution [11]. Knowledge of these mosquito vectors is important for understanding the general epidemiology, transmission cycles, and outbreaks of the disease. Mosquitoes from the *Aedes* genus, in particular, are the primary reservoirs and are essential for the inter-epidemic maintenance and viral transmission of RVFV [1, 11]. Other mosquito species, namely *Culex*, *Anopheles,* and *Mansonia* spp. are considered secondary or amplifying vectors, and they might play a role in the epidemic (epizootic) outbreaks of RVF [11, 17, 18]. The importance of the Aedes mosquitoes is highlighted by the fact that in these mosquitoes transovarial (vertical) transmission takes place to maintain the virus in the mosquito population. The eggs of these Aedine mosquitoes are able to survive prolonged periods of desiccation and are able to successfully hatch following exposure to high rainfall [1, 11, 18]. In this way, mosquito eggs that are infected with RVFV transovarially can yield infected mosquitoes that transmit the disease to susceptible vertebrates, starting a local outbreak. This initial part of the disease outbreak, the enzootic cycle, is often based upon the infection of wildlife hosts [11]. Therefore, some studies have evaluated wildlife populations as potential reservoirs of infection, although this is always a feature of the transmission cycle. Additionally, it is hypothesized that there may be low levels of viral circulation that are not dependent on increased rainfalls as part of this enzootic cycle [11, 18].

Once RVF infection has been established in a susceptible host population, the virus can spread between mammal hosts, and thereafter, the secondary mosquito vectors may begin to transmit and amplify the disease outbreak [17]. This sort of disease pattern is most commonly encountered with domestic livestock (particularly ruminants) and may lead to epizootic spread. The epizootic cycle includes multiple mosquito species, as mentioned, and typically follows a period of high rainfall that has potentiated an increase in mosquito populations, as mosquitoes are able to breed in the filled and flooded pans (vleis) and other water bodies [1, 11, 18]. The epizootic cycle with infection of multiple mosquito and livestock species may cause a surge in RVF cases, which then increases the likelihood of a spillover of disease into humans, which can bring about an epidemic.

In addition to biological transmission, mechanical transmission of the virus by biting flies also contributes to disease spread. The disease can also spread mechanically by fomites and by coming in contact with the blood and tissue of infected animals.

Rift Valley fever disease outbreaks have historically occurred exclusively on the African continent and Arabian Peninsula [1–3]. Some of the most significant outbreaks over the last century were in Kenya, South Africa, Egypt, Saudi Arabia, Somalia, and Tanzania, among others [2]. Studies have demonstrated the presence of RVFV in more than 31 countries, indicating that it is quite widespread in the continent.

Of great concern is evidence of the virus in regions previously thought to be free, such as Turkey, Iran, and Iraq, and the proximity of these countries to Europe [4–7].

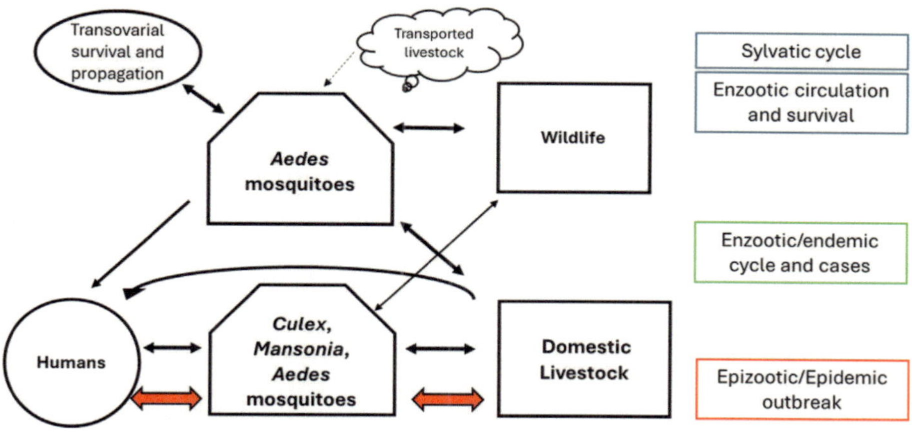

Figure 1.
Diagram illustrating the transmission of RVFV and how different factors fit into (i) enzootic circulation and virus persistence (sylvatic cycle), (ii) enzootic/endemic cycle, (iii) epizootic/epidemic outbreak.

UN subregion	Countries with RVF virus detected or RVFV serological detection	References
Europe	No endemic cases were reported. Suspect cases imported by Armed forces	[9]
Western Asia (Middle East)	Iran*, Iraq*, Jordan*, Saudi Arabia, Türkiye*, Yemen	[1, 2, 4, 5, 7, 19, 20]
Northern Africa	Algeria*, Egypt, Libya*, Sudan, South Sudan, Tunisia*, Western Sahara*	[1, 2, 4, 6, 8, 21]
Western Africa	Burkina Faso, Gambia, Ghana*, Mali, Mauritania, Niger, Nigeria, Senegal	[1, 2, 9, 22–27]
Middle Africa (Central Africa)	Angola, Central African Republic, Cameroon, Chad, Congo, Democratic Republic of Congo, Gabon	[3, 28–35]
Eastern Africa	Comoros, Ethiopia, *East Africa Region*, Kenya, Madagascar, Malawi, Mozambique, Somalia, Tanzania, Uganda, Zambia, Zimbabwe	[1–3, 36–41]
Southern Africa	Botswana, Namibia, South Africa	[1–3, 18, 42]
Other	Mayotte (French overseas department – EU), *Potential imported case to Martinique*, *Imported case to China*	[3, 9, 29, 30]
	*Countries not currently updated on the CDC online RVF distribution map	

Table 1.
Different subregions and countries where rift valley fever has been reported through virus detection, clinical diagnosis, outbreaks, or serological detection (including seroprevalence studies).

One of the factors that makes RVFV a difficult pathogen to track and study for viral presence and distribution is the dependence on the mosquito vectors and rainfall patterns as described. Additionally, the role of animal (wildlife) reservoirs in maintaining subclinical levels of infection in an area is uncertain.

Rift Valley fever virus infects many mammalian species, and as mentioned, wildlife species are important for the transmission and maintenance of the virus. Humans are also susceptible to infection, although historical case numbers in humans are lower than in animals. Infections in humans are frequently associated with vocational risk factors associated with working with animals, which may lead to contact with infected tissues (such as veterinarians or carcass processing) [1, 11]. Infected *Culex* and *Mansonia* mosquitoes can transmit infection to humans, and this vector-based spread accounts for the higher case numbers in outbreak situations [11]. Domestic ruminants are generally the most severely affected animals, with cattle, goats, and sheep being the most widely affected. However, the severity of the disease (pathogenicity) differs between these species, where sheep experience the most severe infection and cattle have the least severe infection of the three species [1, 11, 12]. Furthermore, infection in young animals is typically the worst, and pregnant animals may also be severely affected (**Figure 1** and **Table 1**).

3. Clinical features

Rift Valley Fever virus has a short incubation period of about 3 days in animals. Sheep and goats exhibit similar clinical signs that include fever, inappetence, and nasal discharge, which could be mucopurulent and hemorrhagic diarrhea. The disease can lead to a high rate of abortion, nearing 100% in pregnant ewes that are infected with RVFV, which is often referred to as "abortion storms". The virus causes a mild disease in cattle, and infected cattle show less severe clinical signs. Other animals, such as camels, dogs, and cats, can be affected by RVFV, but the virus typically does not cause any clinical signs except occasionally in young animals.

In livestock, common clinical signs associated with severe disease include icterus, hemorrhagic diarrhea, and respiratory distress or labored breathing [12]. Rift Valley fever virus has significant effects on pregnant animals, where infection at any stage can cause the death of the fetus and abortion [1, 11]. Therefore, abortions and teratogenic effects are common, and abortion storms (widespread abortions) might be seen where flocks or herds are affected and previously unexposed. Mortality rates in animals can be high, ranging from 10 to 50% in adult ruminants, and the highest mortality rate of 90% seen in young lambs [12].

The severity of the disease may also vary in animals, particularly based on the level of previous exposure to RVFV and the level of herd immunity present. In all animals, infection will likely lead to pyrexia and a significant drop in production [43]. Although in younger, naïve, and immune-compromised animals, the disease will likely show more severe signs and lesions, particularly in sheep and goats, and high mortality rates might be seen [1, 11].

In humans, the disease commonly resembles a mild to moderate flu-like illness with pyrexia (often of unknown origin) and body aches [17, 43–45]. The incubation period in humans ranges from 2 to 6 days. The typical clinical signs of hemorrhagic disease include fever, headache, chills, severe muscle pain, and sometimes vomiting and diarrhea. The virus infection in humans is mostly self-limiting, with clinical signs reduced within a week. A small percentage of affected people may develop severe diseases with liver necrosis, renal failure, pneumonia, and meningoencephalitis. Retinitis leading to vision loss is also common in people affected with severe forms of the disease.

4. Pathogenesis and pathology

RVFV is associated with multiple different clinical presentations and disease states in animals and humans. Some of the common features of infection are hepatic damage, viremia, pyrexia, lesions in the gastrointestinal and respiratory tract, disruptions in hemostasis, abortions, and teratogenesis [1, 11, 12]. Following infection, the development of viremia in animals is typically rapid, occurring within hours to days (the most rapid development occurs in neonatal lambs) [43]. The viremia helps to spread the virus diffusely into other target organs and leads to the disease symptoms experienced. The virus replicates in the cytoplasm of infected cells; however, through the NS proteins, the virus forms intranuclear inclusions, which can be seen histologically in infected tissues [16, 46]. These NS proteins are important viral virulence factors, as they disrupt host transcription and reduce innate host antiviral responses [16]. Virus replication is believed to take place in the liver, spleen, lymph nodes, lungs, kidneys, adrenal glands, and less commonly in the brain. It is believed that the lesions seen with RVFV infection are mainly through virus-induced cell and tissue lysis, especially those seen in hepatocytes [43]. However, immunopathological effects leading to some of the tissue damage and symptoms seen are also likely.

Typically, in ruminants, pathological lesions occur in the liver, where hemorrhage and necrosis are common, and may lead to almost pathognomonic lesions in the liver and gall bladder [12, 43]. In addition, there may be necrotic and hemorrhagic lesions in the spleen and gastrointestinal tract, as well as pulmonary congestion.

In humans, severe disease forms involving multiple organ systems may be seen, such as renal failure or ocular lesions, which might lead to partial or complete vision loss [44, 45]. Additionally, in some cases, there may be fatal disease states and complications in humans, such as the development of encephalitis or a hemorrhagic syndrome where necrotic hepatitis may occur [45].

5. Diagnosis and control

RVFV is a disease of global significance, and a lot of attention is being paid to monitoring the viral distribution and spread. Accurate diagnostic assays are essential, and the two main principles of diagnostic tests are the detection of the virus and the detection of associated antibodies. For direct detection of the virus, nucleic acid tests are the most common, and reverse transcription real-time/quantitative polymerase chain reaction (RT-qPCR) is the most common test and provides the highest sensitivity and specificity [1, 47]. However, additional nucleic acid base assays are receiving more attention and may become more common, such as RT-loop mediated amplification (RT-LAMP), recombinase polymerase amplification (RPA), and multiplex PCRs [47–49]. Within these, RT-LAMP and RPA assays offer very high sensitivity through very low limits for viral detection per reaction, and multiplex assays offer convenience and flexibility when testing for multiple agents [47].

Detection of antibodies to RVFV is mainly used to determine viral presence in a region (retrospective) or exposure in animals. These assays generally target either IgM or IgG antibodies, with IgM indicative of a more acute exposure and IgG antibody levels demonstrating exposure to the virus in the past [1, 11, 47]. The most widely used assays are ELISA assays using serum samples, and these can usually be used to test large sample numbers. However, where positive results are detected, the approach is to retest using the gold-standard assay for determining the presence of antibodies, the viral neutralization test (VNT) [19, 47]. While all of these diagnostic assays are primarily lab-based assays, the VNT has historically been carried out in biosafety level 3 laboratories because the RVF virus is used to perform the assay. Besides the use of validated diagnostic assays, one should also keep in mind other epidemiological data such as recent rainfall patterns and environmental conditions, when considering possible cases of RVFV.

There is no defined treatment for RVFV infection other than palliative care and symptom relief. Therefore, control measures should depend on vaccination as well as vector control and other potential environmental control measures, given the importance of mosquitoes in the spread of the disease. Environmental measures that help to reduce mosquito breeding and populations may also help to reduce the spread of the virus from the vectors. Currently, there are no approved vaccines available for use in humans, but multiple vaccines have been used in domestic ruminants for decades. Routine vaccination resulting in herd immunity can help to reduce the high levels of losses and abortions that are seen in naïve flocks and herds and is recommended in endemic areas. Care should, however, be taken as there can be serious side effects when vaccinating pregnant animals (abortions and teratogenicity) with replication-competent vaccines, such as the Smithburn strain vaccine [50–52]. Additionally, vaccination of animals could confuse the interpretation of test results in areas as current vaccines do not facilitate differentiating infected from vaccinated animals (DIVA), and this could be particularly problematic in areas where the status and presence of the virus are uncertain [11, 50].

6. Conclusions

Rift Valley fever is a serious viral disease that affects both humans and animals. The significant history of disease outbreaks and the widespread distribution of cases across and beyond the African continent exemplify the virus's ability to survive and spread beyond previously considered geographical boundaries. Domestic ruminants, particularly sheep, are the most severely affected animals by RVF outbreaks, and in naïve populations, the losses can be devastating. Additionally, RVF epizootics bring an increased risk for disease spillover to people, especially where there is a close livestock-human interface. Intervention should focus on prevention strategies, where routine livestock vaccination is encouraged, and vector control may also help to reduce the further spread of the virus. In the event of a disease outbreak, rapid and accurate diagnosis, as provided by RT-qPCR, is valuable for facilitating an effective response. Coupled with the expanded distribution of mosquitoes globally and the effects of climate change, RVFV is an emerging zoonotic pathogen of concern in different parts of the world. The development of better molecular diagnostic tools, including point-of-care tests such as RT-LAMP, as well as development of effective preventive measures, including vaccines for use in humans, needs to be further explored.

Acknowledgements

The authors thankfully acknowledge the help and support of faculty and staff at the Athens Veterinary Diagnostic Laboratory, University of Georgia, Athens, GA.

Conflict of interest

The authors declare no conflict of interest.

Author details

Binu T. Velayudhan* and Shaun van den Hurk
Athens Veterinary Diagnostic Laboratory, University of Georgia, Athens, GA, United States of America

*Address all correspondence to: binu.velayudhan@uga.edu

IntechOpen

© 2024 The Author(s). Licensee IntechOpen. This chapter is distributed under the terms of the Creative Commons Attribution License (http://creativecommons.org/licenses/by/4.0), which permits unrestricted use, distribution, and reproduction in any medium, provided the original work is properly cited.

References

[1] Wright D et al. Rift valley fever: Biology and epidemiology. The Journal of General Virology. 2019;**100**(8):1187-1199

[2] Kenawy MA, Abdel-Hamid YM, Beier JC. Rift valley fever in Egypt and other African countries: Historical review, recent outbreaks and possibility of disease occurrence in Egypt. Acta Tropica. 2018;**181**:40-49

[3] Clark MHA et al. Systematic literature review of rift valley fever virus seroprevalence in livestock, wildlife and humans in Africa from 1968 to 2016. PLoS Neglected Tropical Diseases. 2018;**12**(7):e0006627

[4] Nielsen SS et al. Rift valley fever - epidemiological update and risk of introduction into Europe. EFSA Journal. 2020;**18**(3):e06041

[5] Fakour S, Naserabadi S, Ahmadi E. A serological and hematological study on rift valley fever and associated risk factors in aborted sheep at Kurdistan province in west of Iran. Comparative Immunology, Microbiology and Infectious Diseases. 2021;**75**:101620

[6] Selmi R et al. First serological evidence of the rift valley fever phlebovirus in Tunisian camels. Acta Tropica. 2020;**207**:105462

[7] Gür S et al. The first serological evidence for rift valley fever infection in the camel, goitered gazelle and Anatolian water buffaloes in Turkey. Tropical Animal Health and Production. 2017;**49**(7):1531-1535

[8] Di Nardo A et al. Evidence of rift valley fever seroprevalence in the Sahrawi semi-nomadic pastoralist system, Western Sahara. BMC Veterinary Research. 2014;**10**(1):92

[9] Tong C et al. Tracking rift valley fever: From Mali to Europe and other countries, 2016. Euro Surveillance. 2019;**24**(8):1-9

[10] Sasaya T et al. ICTV virus taxonomy profile: Phenuiviridae 2023: This article is part of the ICTV virus taxonomy profiles collection. Journal of General Virology. 2023;**104**:1-2

[11] Hartman A. Rift valley fever. Clinics in Laboratory Medicine. 2017;**37**(2):285-301

[12] Nair N et al. Rift valley fever virus–Infection, pathogenesis and host immune responses. Pathogens. 2023;**12**(9):1174

[13] Wichgers Schreur PJ et al. Four-segmented rift valley fever virus induces sterile immunity in sheep after a single vaccination. Vaccine. 2015;**33**(12):1459-1464

[14] Alkan C, Jurado-Cobena E, Ikegami T. Advancements in rift valley fever vaccines: A historical overview and prospects for next generation candidates. npj Vaccines. 2023;**8**(1):171

[15] Fatima I et al. Designing of a multi-epitopes-based peptide vaccine against rift valley fever virus and its validation through integrated computational approaches. Computers in Biology and Medicine. 2022;**141**:105151

[16] Ikegami T, Makino S. The pathogenesis of rift valley fever. Viruses. 2011;**3**(5):493-519

[17] McMillen CM, Hartman AL. Rift valley fever in animals and humans: Current perspectives. Antiviral Research. 2018;**156**:29-37

[18] Rissmann M et al. Mechanisms of inter-epidemic maintenance of rift valley fever phlebovirus. Antiviral Research. 2020;**174**:104692

[19] Wichgers Schreur PJ et al. A novel highly sensitive, rapid and safe rift valley fever virus neutralization test. Journal of Virological Methods. 2017;**248**:26-30

[20] Obaidat MM et al. Rift valley fever and Crimean-Congo hemorrhagic fever viruses in ruminants, Jordan. Emerging Infectious Diseases. 2021;**27**(2):653-655

[21] Trabelsi MK et al. Serological evidence of rift valley fever viral infection among camels imported into southern Algeria. Comparative Immunology, Microbiology and Infectious Diseases. 2023;**100**:102035

[22] Tinto B et al. Rift valley fever in West Africa: A zoonotic disease with multiple socio-economic consequences. One Health. 2023;**17**:100583

[23] Subudhi S et al. Seroprevalence of rift valley fever virus antibodies in cattle in Mali, 2005-2014. The American Journal of Tropical Medicine and Hygiene. 2018;**98**(3):872-874

[24] Adamu AM et al. Risk factors for rift valley fever virus seropositivity in one-humped camels (Camelus dromedarius) and pastoralist knowledge and practices in northern Nigeria. One Health. 2021;**13**:100340

[25] Adamu AM et al. Serosurvey on sheep unravel circulation of rift valley fever virus in Nigeria. EcoHealth. 2020;**17**(3):393-397

[26] Olaleye OD, Tomori O, Schmitz H. Rift valley fever in Nigeria: Infections in domestic animals. Revue Scientifique et Technique. 1996;**15**(3):937-946

[27] Lagare A et al. First occurrence of rift valley fever outbreak in Niger, 2016. Veterinary Medicine and Science. 2019;**5**(1):70-78

[28] Özcelik R et al. Seroprevalence and associated risk factors of brucellosis, rift valley fever and Q fever among settled and mobile agro-pastoralist communities and their livestock in Chad. PLoS Neglected Tropical Diseases. 2023;**17**(6):e0011395

[29] Bob NS et al. Detection of rift valley fever virus lineage H from South Africa through the syndromic sentinel surveillance network in Senegal. Open Forum Infectious Diseases. 2022;**9**(3):ofab655

[30] Liu J et al. The first imported case of rift valley fever in China reveals a genetic reassortment of different viral lineages. Emerging Microbes & Infections. 2017;**6**(1):1-7

[31] Tshilenge GM et al. Rift valley fever virus in small ruminants in the Democratic Republic of the Congo. The Onderstepoort Journal of Veterinary Research. 2019;**86**(1):e1-e5

[32] Mbanzulu KM et al. Mosquito-borne viruses circulating in Kinshasa, Democratic Republic of the Congo. International Journal of Infectious Diseases. 2017;**57**:32-37

[33] Becquart P et al. Evidence for circulation of rift valley fever virus in wildlife and domestic animals in a forest environment in Gabon, Central Africa. PLoS Neglected Tropical Diseases. 2024;**18**(3):e0011756

[34] Sado FY et al. Seroprevalence of rift valley fever virus in domestic ruminants of various origins in two markets of Yaoundé, Cameroon. PLoS Neglected Tropical Diseases. 2022;**16**(8):e0010683

[35] Gonzalez JP et al. Antibody prevalence against haemorrhagic fever viruses in randomized representative central African populations. Research in Virology. 1989;**140**:319-331

[36] Ibrahim M et al. Sero-prevalence of brucellosis, Q-fever and rift valley fever in humans and livestock in Somali region, Ethiopia. PLoS Neglected Tropical Diseases. 2021;**15**(1):e0008100

[37] Rugarabamu S et al. Seroprevalence and associated risk factors of selected zoonotic viral hemorrhagic fevers in Tanzania. International Journal of Infectious Diseases. 2021;**109**:174-181

[38] Tumusiime D et al. Participatory survey of risk factors and pathways for rift valley fever in pastoral and agropastoral communities of Uganda. Preventive Veterinary Medicine. 2023;**221**:106071

[39] Lysholm S et al. Seropositivity rates of zoonotic pathogens in small ruminants and associated public health risks at informal urban markets in Zambia. Acta Tropica. 2022;**225**:106217

[40] Kainga H et al. Seroprevalence and associated risk factors of rift valley fever in livestock from three ecological zones of Malawi. Pathogens. 2022;**11**(11):1349

[41] Fafetine JM et al. Rift valley fever outbreak in livestock, Mozambique, 2014. Emerging Infectious Diseases. 2016;**22**(12):2165-2167

[42] Thompson P et al. Co-circulation of rift valley fever virus and other zoonotic arboviruses at the human-livestock-wildlife interface in KwaZulu-Natal, South Africa. International Journal of Infectious Diseases. 2020;**101**:535

[43] Coetzer JAW et al. Rift valley fever. In: Coetzer JAW et al., editors. Infectious Diseases of Livestock. South Africa: Anipedia; 2021

[44] Anywaine Z et al. Clinical manifestations of rift valley fever in humans: Systematic review and meta-analysis. PLoS Neglected Tropical Diseases. 2022;**16**(3):e0010233

[45] Javelle E et al. The challenging management of rift valley fever in humans: Literature review of the clinical disease and algorithm proposal. Annals of Clinical Microbiology and Antimicrobials. 2020;**19**(1):4

[46] Struthers JK, Swanepoel R. Identification of a major non-structural protein in the nuclei of rift valley fever virus-infected cells. The Journal of General Virology. 1982;**60**(Pt. 2):381-384

[47] Lapa D et al. Rift valley fever virus: An overview of the current status of diagnostics. Biomedicines. 2024;**12**(3):540

[48] Yao Y et al. A self-powered rapid loading microfluidic chip for vector-borne viruses detection using RT-LAMP. Sensors and Actuators B: Chemical. 2021;**333**:129521

[49] Choi Y, Kim Y. Application of multiplex realtime PCR detection for hemorrhagic fever syndrome viruses. Journal of Infection and Public Health. 2023;**16**(12):1933-1941

[50] Kitandwe PK et al. An overview of rift valley fever vaccine development strategies. Vaccines. 2022;**10**(11):1794

[51] Smithburn KC. Rift valley fever; the neurotropic adaptation of the virus and the experimental use of this modified virus as a vaccine. British

Journal of Experimental Pathology. 1949;**30**(1):1-16

[52] Matsiela MS et al. Safety and immunogenicity of inactivated rift valley fever Smithburn viral vaccine in sheep. Virology Journal. 2023;**20**(1):221

Chapter 5

The Evolution of African Swine Fever: Past, Present, and Future Perspectives

Sandra Barroso-Arévalo and Cristina Jurado-Díaz

Abstract

African swine fever (ASF) poses a major threat to global swine health, impacting agriculture and food security worldwide. This chapter reviews the historical context, current challenges, and future prospects of the disease. It highlights the significant economic losses caused by ASF outbreaks and emphasizes the need for strict biosecurity measures, culling policies, and trade restrictions. The epidemiology of ASF is discussed in detail, covering its transmission cycles involving domestic pigs, wild suids, and soft ticks of the genus *Ornithodoros*. The African swine fever virus (ASFV) utilizes complex mechanisms to evade the immune system, complicating vaccine development. The chapter also reviews current diagnostic techniques, from traditional to advanced molecular and serological methods, stressing the importance of rapid and accurate detection. The immune response to ASFV is explored, focusing on innate and adaptive immunity, which is a key to developing effective vaccines. Various vaccine strategies are discussed, particularly live attenuated vaccines (LAVs), their potential, and associated safety concerns. The chapter concludes by emphasizing the need for continued research, innovation, and international collaboration to mitigate the impact of ASF on the swine industry. It aims to enhance understanding of ASF and inform strategies for its control and prevention.

Keywords: African swine fever virus, epidemiology, vaccines, immune response, disease management, swine health

1. Introduction

African swine fever (ASF) has emerged as a critical issue in global swine health, posing a significant threat to agriculture worldwide. This highly contagious viral disease affects both domestic and wild swine. Virulent strains often lead to mortality rates nearing 100% [1]. It is important to note that ASF is non-zoonotic in that it is not spread to humans. Beyond its impact on animal health, ASF brings substantial economic losses to the pig farming industry, disrupts pork supply chains, and severely affects rural communities that rely on pig farming. The swine industry worldwide faces numerous challenges due to ASF outbreaks, including stringent biosecurity measures, stamping out policies, and trade restrictions on pig and pork products.

These necessary measures to control the disease lead to economic hardship for farmers, increased pork prices, and food insecurity in affected regions [2, 3].

This chapter aims to provide a comprehensive overview of ASF's evolution, examining its historical context, current challenges, and future prospects. We will explore the origins and spread of ASF, detail significant outbreaks that have shaped our current understanding and responses, and discuss contemporary strategies for diagnosing, controlling, and preventing ASF. Additionally, we will look at future scientific and policy advancements that could influence ASF management, focusing on vaccine development.

2. History of ASF

ASF traces its roots back to Africa, where the disease was first identified. The disease likely originated in a sylvatic cycle involving wild African suids, particularly warthogs, and soft ticks of the genus *Ornithodoros*, which serve as vectors and reservoirs. The first reported outbreak of ASF occurred in Kenya in 1921, marking the beginning of our understanding of this devastating disease [4]. The causative agent, African swine fever virus (ASFV), is a large, double-stranded DNA virus belonging to the *Asfarviridae* family. Structurally, ASFV is complex, featuring an icosahedral capsid surrounded by multiple lipid membranes, which contribute to its stability and resilience in various environments. The viral genome, approximately 170–190 kilobases in size, encodes over 150 proteins, many of which are involved in the virus's ability to evade the host immune system. ASFV is highly variable, with 24 known genotypes identified based on the B646L gene encoding the p72 protein [5, 6]. Immunologically, ASFV presents a formidable challenge due to its sophisticated mechanisms for immune evasion, including the inhibition of host cell apoptosis and modulation of the host immune response. The virus's ability to persist in host tissues and evade immune detection complicates the development of effective vaccines, making ASFV a persistent and difficult pathogen to control [3, 7].

Initially, ASF was largely confined to Africa, where it remained endemic for several decades. Sporadic outbreaks occurred in domestic pig populations, often linked to contact with wild suids or ticks. These early outbreaks highlighted the urgent need for improved understanding and control measures to prevent the disease's spread. The situation changed dramatically in the late 1950s when ASF spread beyond Africa for the first time. In 1957, ASF was introduced to Portugal where it was eradicated rapidly. In 1960, the virus escaped for the second time from Africa to Portugal, marking the beginning of its establishment in Europe. The disease quickly spread to neighboring Spain, where it remained endemic for decades. Moreover, another 9 countries were affected by ASF, namely, France, Italy, Malta, Belgium, the Netherlands, Cuba, Brazil, the Dominican Republic, and Haiti. The disease was eradicated from all these countries except from the Italian island of Sardinia (endemic since 1978) [3, 7].

In the early 2000s, ASF re-emerged as a major threat with a severe outbreak in Georgia in 2007. This outbreak marked the beginning of a new, more aggressive phase of ASF spread. From Georgia (2007), the virus quickly spread to Armenia (2007), the Russian Federation (2007), Ukraine (2012), and Belarus (2013). The spread in Eastern Europe affected both domestic pig and wild boar populations, complicating control efforts. The situation escalated further in the mid-2010s when ASF spread through the Baltic region and Eastern Europe. Countries such as Poland (2014), Lithuania (2014), Latvia (2014), Estonia (2014), Moldova (2016), Czech Republic (2017), Romania (2017), Hungary (2018), Bulgaria (2018), Belgium (2018), Eslovaquia (2019), Serbia (2019), Greece (2020), Germany (2020), North Macedonia (2022), Italy (2022), Croatia (2023), Bosnia and Herzegovina (2023), Sweden (2023), Kosovo (2023), Montenegro (2024), and Albania (2024) have reported outbreaks in domestic pigs and/or wild boar. So far, 25 countries and territories have notified the presence of ASF. The affected European Union member states have reported 85% of cases of wild boar (excluding Romania from this analysis). This period saw a significant increase in the number of outbreaks and substantial economic losses due to the culling of infected and at-risk animals and the imposition of trade restrictions [3, 7].

One of the most devastating outbreaks in recent history occurred in China in 2018. As the world's largest producer and consumer of pork, China faced unprecedented challenges as ASF spread rapidly across the country. Millions of pigs were culled to contain the virus, leading to a significant reduction in pork production and a subsequent increase in global pork prices. The outbreak in China had far-reaching implications, highlighting the global nature of the ASF threat and the need for coordinated international efforts to manage the disease. The rapid spread of ASF in Asia did not stop in China.

So far, 19 neighboring Asian countries and territories, including Mongolia (2019), Vietnam (2019), Cambodia (2019), Hong Kong (2019), North and South Korea (2019), Laos (2019), the Philippines (2019), Myanmar (2019), Indonesia (2019), Timor-Leste (2019), India (2020), Malaysia (2021), Butan (2021), Thailand (2021), Nepal (2022), Bangladesh (2023), and Singapur (2023), also reported outbreaks. The extensive spread of ASF in Asia underscored the virus's resilience and adaptability, as well as the challenges inherent in controlling a disease that can spread through various routes, including direct contact between pigs, contaminated feed and equipment, and wild boar populations. ASF has made its way to new regions, including Oceania and the Caribbean. In 2020, Papua New Guinea notified outbreaks of ASF in domestic pigs. In 2021, the Dominican Republic and Haiti reported outbreaks, marking the first known presence of ASF in the Americas in several decades. This development has raised concerns about the potential spread of ASF to other countries in the Western Hemisphere, prompting increased vigilance and biosecurity measures to prevent further dissemination [8–10].

Throughout its history, ASF has demonstrated an alarming ability to spread across continents, impacting both domestic and wild pig populations. Its persistence and adaptability, combined with the difficulties of controlling its spread in various agricultural systems and environments, make ASF one of the toughest challenges the global swine industry faces today [11].

3. Epidemiology and control of ASF

Today, ASF is found across multiple continents, affecting countries in Africa, Europe, Asia, Oceania, and the Americas. The disease's spread and maintenance are facilitated by various epidemiological cycles: the domestic pig cycle, the sylvatic cycle, and the tick-pig cycle [12]. In the domestic pig cycle, ASF spreads rapidly through direct and indirect contact between infected and susceptible pigs, as well as through the consumption of pork products, food waste, contaminated feed, equipment, vehicles, and clothing. The sylvatic cycle involves wild suids, such as warthogs, bushpigs, and soft ticks [13, 14]. These soft ticks belong to the genus *Ornithodoros*, specifically to the *O. moubata* complex. Wild suids can harbor and replicate the virus but show no clinical signs [15]. The pig-tick cycle has been reported in Africa and Europe [16]. In Portugal and Spain, ASFV was transmitted in certain areas by *O. erraticus* soft ticks. These soft ticks act as vectors, maintaining and spreading the virus within pig populations. Moreover, they can remain infected for long periods, making them a persistent source of ASFV [17, 18]. In addition to this, interactions in wildlife interfaces can facilitate transmission. It may occur between domestic pigs and wild boar and vice versa, as well as within wild boar populations. Such contacts can be among live individuals, their carcasses, or vector-borne transmission [11].

Several factors contribute to the persistence and propagation of ASF. The virus's ability to survive in various environmental conditions, including within meat and carcasses, enhances its spread [19–21]. Inadequate biosecurity measures, particularly in small-scale and backyard farms, facilitate the virus's transmission. Furthermore, human activities, such as the movement of pigs and pork products, play a significant role in the disease's dissemination [2, 22]. The presence of ASF in wild boar populations also complicates control efforts, as these animals can move across borders and spread the virus over wide areas [23–25].

The socioeconomic impact of ASF is profound, particularly for pig producers. The disease leads to substantial economic losses due to the death of infected pigs, the culling of at-risk animals, and the costs associated with implementing control measures. These economic burdens are especially heavy for smallholder farmers who lack the resources to invest in comprehensive biosecurity measures [26, 27]. ASF also affects food supplies and the livelihoods of rural communities that depend on pig farming. In regions heavily reliant on pork as a primary protein source, ASF outbreaks can lead to significant food shortages and increased prices for pork products. This situation exacerbates poverty and food insecurity, particularly in low- and middle-income countries where pig farming is a vital part of the agricultural economy [28]. ASFV does not pose any risk to human health but control measures imply the destruction of any potentially contaminated meat or pork products.

Effective control and prevention of ASF require a multifaceted approach, combining biosecurity measures, culling policies, movement restrictions, and surveillance. Implementing strict biosecurity protocols on pig farms is essential to prevent the introduction and spread of ASFV. These measures include controlling access to farms, disinfecting vehicles and equipment, and ensuring that feed and water are free from contamination. Culling infected and at-risk animals is a critical component of ASF control. While this measure is often necessary to prevent the spread of the virus, it is economically and emotionally devastating for farmers. To minimize the impact, it is crucial to provide adequate compensation to affected farmers and to implement culling humanely and efficiently. Movement restrictions on pigs and pork products are also vital in controlling ASF. These restrictions help prevent the spread of the virus to new areas and reduce the risk of outbreaks. International collaboration and compliance with trade regulations are essential to ensure the effectiveness of these measures. Additionally, public awareness campaigns, aimed at educating hunters and the general populace, are indispensable for fostering a collective responsibility toward containment efforts in wild boar populations. Surveillance and monitoring are indispensable for early detection and response to ASF outbreaks. Robust surveillance systems, including regular testing and reporting, help track the disease's spread and inform control strategies. International collaboration, such as that facilitated by the World Organization for Animal Health (WOAH) and the Food and Agriculture Organization (FAO), is crucial in coordinating global surveillance efforts and sharing best practices [1–3, 22, 29].

Accurate and timely diagnosis is crucial for controlling ASF [30, 31]. Diagnostic techniques have evolved significantly, moving from traditional methods to advanced technologies. Initially, ASF diagnosis relied on clinical signs and post-mortem examinations, which, while indicative, lacked specificity and sensitivity. Today, molecular diagnostics, particularly real-time polymerase chain reaction (PCR) assays, are the gold standard for ASF detection. PCR allows for the rapid and precise identification of ASFV DNA in blood, tissue, and a wide range of samples and matrixes. This method is highly sensitive and specific making it indispensable for early detection and outbreak management. However, the viability of the detected virus should be determined by isolating ASFV in primary cell culture.

The use of serological techniques, such as ELISA (Enzyme-Linked Immunosorbent Assay) and immunoblotting, is an important tool for diagnosing ASF. If infected animals do not die from the acute phase of the disease, they can develop large quantities of specific antibodies. Vaccines that do not distinguish between infected and vaccinated animals are currently being used in Vietnam and neighboring regions. This complicates the interpretation of serological tests, as it becomes impossible to determine the source of the antibodies. Other diagnostic methods [32–36], such as loop-mediated isothermal amplification (LAMP), and recombinase polymerase amplification (RPA), among others, are also being developed and implemented. Some of them provide a quick, field-deployable means of detecting ASFV, making them useful in remote areas with limited laboratory infrastructure. Although less sensitive than PCR, their ease of use and rapid results make them valuable for initial screening during outbreaks. These techniques offer the potential for rapid, on-site ASF detection, further enhancing disease management capabilities.

4. Immune response to ASFV

The immune system plays a crucial role during viral infections, being the first line of defense of the organism, and it will determine the process outcome. Understanding the immune response in the case of ASFV is critical to developing effective control and prevention strategies. The immune system comprises innate and adaptive responses [37]. The innate immune system is the first line of defense, providing an instant and non-specific response to pathogens through cells like macrophages and dendritic cells [38]. The adaptive immune system provides a specific defense through lymphocytes, which include B cells that secrete antibodies and T cells that destroy infected cells. Both are essential in the ASFV immune response. ASFV can weaken the immune response by directly infecting macrophages and dendritic cells, hindering their ability to activate other immune cells and produce antiviral molecules. While this interaction and compression are so important to the development of the vaccine, the evasion mechanisms of ASFV are highly developed, and, therefore, the virus can avoid the host defense mechanisms [39]. The first route silenced by ASFV is the cGAS-STING pathway, a major player in recognizing pathogen DNA and activating an immune response. The cGAS detects viral DNA in the cytoplasm to synthesize cyclic GMP-AMP (cGAMP) for further activation of STING. Subsequently, the signaling molecule STING activates a signaling pathway that activates type I interferons and other pro-inflammatory cytokines important for antiviral defense. Several proteins encoded by ASFV have been shown to inhibit this pathway so that detection can be avoided. For instance, proteins pC129R and pEP364R bind cGAS directly, thus inhibiting it from interacting with DNA to synthesize cGAMP. Other proteins of ASFV inhibit the nuclear import of interferon regulatory factor 3 (IRF3), an important transcription factor, hence further stopping the production of type I interferons [38].

Another critical pathway ASFV manipulates is the NF-κB signaling pathway, crucial for the pro-inflammatory response to infections. Upon activation by pattern recognition receptors (PRRs) detecting viral components, NF-κB translocates to the nucleus and induces the expression of genes involved in inflammation and immune responses. ASFV proteins such as pD345L and pI226R inhibit this pathway by blocking the activity of IκB kinase (IKK), preventing the degradation of IκB and subsequent activation of NF-κB. By dampening NF-κB signaling, ASFV diminishes the host's inflammatory response, aiding in immune evasion and viral persistence [40]. Additionally, ASFV ensures the survival of infected cells by inhibiting apoptosis, or programmed cell death, which is a vital mechanism by which infected cells can limit viral replication and spread. ASFV encodes several proteins that inhibit apoptosis, ensuring the survival of infected cells. The protein A179L, a homolog of the B-cell lymphoma 2 (Bcl-2) family, binds to and neutralizes pro-apoptotic proteins, preventing the initiation of apoptosis. Another ASFV protein, A224L, blocks the activation of caspase-3, a key enzyme in the apoptotic pathway, thereby promoting cell survival. Through these mechanisms, ASFV ensures the continued viability of infected cells, facilitating ongoing viral replication [41].

All these molecular mechanisms trigger the disruption of host cellular and humoral immune responses, by impairing the functions of key immune cells, such as monocytes, macrophages, and dendritic cells, and interfering with antigen-antibody binding, significantly affecting the host's ability to develop an effective and adaptive immune response [38]. Monocytes, macrophages, and dendritic cells are the primary antigen-presenting cells (APCs) in the host, playing a crucial role in initiating and regulating the consequent immune responses. Infection of APCs by ASFV leads to differential expression of key cytokines and cell surface markers, impeding their function [42]. For example, infection with the ASFV-Georgia 2007 strain inhibits major cellular immune processes, including MHC class II-mediated antigen processing, M1 macrophage activation, and macrophage autophagy and apoptosis [43–45]. Attenuated ASFV isolates such as BA71V and NH/P68 suppress the expression of MHC class I molecules on infected macrophages, contrasting with more virulent strains. This downregulation impairs macrophage function, reducing their antimicrobial and antiviral activities [46, 47].

Dendritic cells (DCs), specialized APCs, detect, process, and present antigens to lymphocytes. *In vivo* experiments have shown that infection with highly virulent ASFV strains significantly reduces the number of DCs in lymph nodes, hindering the adaptive immune response [48]. Studies with monocyte-derived DCs (MoDCs) infected with different ASFV genotypes revealed that attenuated strains could suppress MHC class I expression, potentially leading to NK cell activation and protection against the virus. ASFV infection also leads to poor cellular immune responses and enhanced lymphocyte apoptosis, causing lymphocytopenia [38, 42, 49]. Cytotoxic T cells, especially CD8+ T cells, play a critical role in the immune response against ASFV. Infections with highly virulent ASFV strains reduce the numbers and functional capacity of these T cells, including decreased perforin expression and a reduction in CD4+ T cells in peripheral blood [49, 50]. The cytotoxicity mediated by NK cells and CD8+ T cells has been associated with immune protection against ASFV, as evidenced by increased NK cell activity and CD8+ cell counts in immunized pigs. Despite the induction of T-effector cells in vaccinated pigs, complete protection remains elusive. Cross-protection provided by attenuated ASFV is correlated with cell-mediated immunity parameters, yet, efficient protection solely through cell-mediated responses has proven challenging [42, 46]. Cytokines and chemokines are also involved in the regulation of the immune response. The induction of pro-inflammatory cytokines like IL-1β, IL-6, and TNF-α, and anti-inflammatory cytokines like IL-10 is controlled by the virus at some stages. The balance between these cytokines is required for an effective immune response. Therefore, ASFV modulates cytokine production to evade the immune response. By inhibiting the production of pro-inflammatory cytokines and promoting anti-inflammatory cytokines, ASFV creates an environment conducive to viral replication and persistence [42, 51, 52].

Comprehensive strategies that enhance both humoral and cellular immunity are essential for developing effective ASFV vaccines. In addition, understanding and overcoming these adaptive immune evasion mechanisms are critical for advancing vaccine development and achieving robust protection against ASFV.

5. Current knowledge of vaccine development

The development of an effective vaccine against ASFV is of great importance due to the devastating impact of the disease on global swine health and the associated economic losses. The need for a vaccine that can prevent the spread of ASFV is critical to protect the swine industry and ensure sustainable pork supply chains [53, 54]. Efforts to develop a vaccine against ASFV have been ongoing since the mid-1960s, employing various approaches such as inactivated vaccines, subunit vaccines, DNA vaccines, virus-vectored vaccines, and live attenuated vaccines (LAVs). Historically, inactivated vaccines were among the first tested against ASFV. However, they consistently failed to induce a robust cellular immune response, which seems to be essential for protection against ASFV. Subunit vaccines use specific viral proteins or antigens to elicit an immune response without introducing the entire virus. This approach enhances safety by avoiding risks associated with live or inactivated virus particles. Several ASFV proteins have been identified as potential candidates for subunit vaccines, including p54, p30, pp220, pp62, p72, EP153R, D117L, and CD2v. However, studies have evaluated the immunogenicity of these proteins, showing varying but lower degrees of success. DNA vaccines involve directly inoculating genetic material encoding viral antigens into host cells, which then produce the antigens and stimulate an immune response [55]. In the context of ASFV, DNA vaccines encoding genes such as p54/E183L and p30/CP204L have been explored; however, they have not yet achieved complete protection in vaccinated pigs. Virus-vectored vaccines use a non-replicative viral vector to deliver ASFV antigens to the host [56]. Examples of vectors used include modified vaccinia Ankara (MVA) and adenovirus. Preclinical studies have demonstrated that virus-vectored vaccines can stimulate the production of interferon-gamma (IFN-γ) and specific antibodies, but not full protection [57].

Live attenuated vaccines (LAVs) involve using a weakened form of the virus that can replicate but causes minimal to no disease. These vaccines aim to induce a strong and lasting immune response by closely mimicking natural infection. The use of LAVs derived from naturally occurring virulent strains has been limited, primarily to the experience accumulated in Portugal and Spain during the 1960s [58]. During this period, a large number of animals were vaccinated with LAVs under field conditions, where they were exposed to multiple infections and reinfections with circulating field strain viruses via various routes, likely including contact with infected soft ticks. These vaccinations under field conditions led to the emergence of chronic forms of the disease [59]. In fact, in the field trial conducted in Spain, some animals exhibited chronic clinical signs. Currently, these vaccines have fallen into disuse primarily due to safety concerns arising from their inherent infectious nature [60]. For these reasons, new approaches have been developed to reduce these limitations.

New LAVs have been developed by targeting genes that are crucial for the virus's ability to cause disease. The deletion of these genes renders the virus less virulent or completely attenuated while retaining its ability to elicit a strong immune response [61]. There are three primary strategies for developing LAVs: (1) naturally attenuated strains that exhibit low virulence. However, they often cause chronic or persistent infections and can lead to adverse effects such as skin lesions and joint swelling; (2) serial passage in cell culture: this method involves repeatedly passing the virus through non-natural host cells, such as Vero cells, to attenuate it. While this can reduce virulence, it often leads to a loss of the virus's ability to confer immunity; and (3) gene-deleted strains: this strategy involves the rational deletion of specific virulence genes from the ASFV genome. This is considered the most promising approach due to its ability to produce a safe and effective virus.

LAVs have shown considerable promise in providing effective immunity against ASFV. One example is the ASFV-G-ΔI177L vaccine, developed by the United States Department of Agriculture and tested in Vietnam, which has demonstrated efficacy in protecting pigs against virulent ASFV strains [62]. Studies have shown that this vaccine can induce antibody-mediated immune responses and confer protection against subsequent ASFV challenges. Similarly, the Lv17/WB/Rie1 strain, a naturally attenuated virus isolated from a wild boar in Latvia, has emerged as a good candidate for creating MLV vaccines [63, 64]. This non-hemadsorbent, attenuated genotype II strain has shown robust protection against virulent ASFV isolates in both domestic pigs [49] and wild boar [51, 65], marking it as a promising base for developing deletion mutants that address concerns about reversion to virulence [66]. Another promising vaccine candidate is BA71ΔCD2, based on a live attenuated virus in which the CD2v protein of the parental virulent BA71 strain has been deleted. This prototype has shown potential cross-protection capabilities [46].

LAVs work by stimulating both the humoral (antibody-mediated) and cellular (T-cell-mediated) factors of the immune system [53]. Upon vaccination, the attenuated virus enters the host and begins to replicate, allowing for continuous production of viral antigens necessary to stimulate the immune system. The innate immune system first detects the virus through APCs such as macrophages and DCs. These cells recognize the viral components and trigger the production of cytokines and interferons, which initiate the immune response. APCs process and present viral antigens on their surface using MHC molecules, essential for T cell activation [67]. The adaptive immune response triggered by LAVs involves T helper cells (CD4+) recognizing antigens presented by MHC class II molecules on APCs, leading to their activation and proliferation. These T helper cells release cytokines that activate B cells and cytotoxic T cells. B cells differentiate into plasma cells, producing antibodies that neutralize the virus. Cytotoxic T cells (CD8+), activated by MHC class I molecules, destroy infected cells, reducing viral replication and spread. A significant advantage of LAVs is their ability to induce immunological memory. Memory B cells and T cells generated during the primary immune response provide rapid and robust protection upon subsequent exposure to the virus. This comprehensive immune activation leads to strong and long-lasting immunity, making LAVs more effective than other vaccine approaches. However, LAVs must be carefully monitored for safety, as there is a risk of the virus reverting to a virulent form [68]. Ensuring genetic stability and conducting thorough safety testing are crucial. Despite these challenges, LAVs offer a promising strategy for controlling ASFV, providing robust protection, and preventing disease transmission within pig populations.

6. Conclusions

ASF poses a severe threat to global swine health and the agricultural economy due to its high mortality rates and significant economic impacts. Tracing its history from its origins in Africa to its spread across continents, ASF has shown its persistence and adaptability, causing devastating outbreaks worldwide. The virus's sophisticated mechanisms to evade the immune system and its resilience in various environments make controlling ASF particularly challenging.

Addressing ASF requires a comprehensive approach, combining an improved understanding of its epidemiology, stringent biosecurity measures, and robust surveillance and diagnostic protocols. The development of vaccines, especially LAVs, offers hope for long-lasting immunity. However, ensuring the safety and genetic stability of these vaccines is crucial to prevent them from becoming virulent again. Ultimately, a coordinated strategy involving biosecurity, vaccination, and international collaboration is essential to manage and mitigate ASF's impact. Ongoing research and innovation, coupled with global cooperation, are vital for advancing our capacity to control this devastating disease and protecting the future of the swine industry. The progress made in understanding ASF and developing effective vaccines provides a strong foundation for continued efforts to combat this significant threat.

Acknowledgements

We would like to express our gratitude to all the members of the SUAT group. They are not only exceptional scientists but also wonderful individuals. We are also deeply thankful to the VISAVET and CISA-INIA-CSIC centers for their invaluable support and resources. A special thanks to the VACDIVA project (Grant Agreement ID: 862874. DOI: 10.3030/862874), whose funding has been instrumental in Sandra Barroso-Arévalo's work.

Conflict of interest

The authors declare no conflict of interest.

Acronyms and abbreviations

ASF	African swine fever
ASFV	African swine fever virus
APCs	antigen-presenting cells

cGAMP	cGMP-AMP
DCs	Dendritic cells
dsDNA	Double-stranded DNA
ELISA	Enzyme-Linked Immunosorbent Assay
EU	European Union
FAO	food and agriculture organization
IRF3	interferon regulatory factor 3
ICTV	international committee on taxonomy of viruses
LAMP	loop-mediated isothermal amplification
MHC	major histocompatibility complex
MVA	Modified vaccinia Ankara
MoDCs	Monocyte-derived dendritic cells
O. moubata	*Ornithodoros moubata*
PCR	Polymerase chain reaction
RPA	Recombinase polymerase amplification
CD4+	T-helper cells
TNF-α	Tumor necrosis factor alpha
WOAH	World Organization for Animal Health

Author details

Sandra Barroso-Arévalo[1]* and Cristina Jurado-Díaz[2]

1 Complutense University of Madrid, VISAVET Center, Madrid, Spain

2 Centro de Investigación en Sanidad Animal, Instituto Nacional de Investigación y Tecnología Agraria y Alimentaria, Consejo Superior de Investigaciones Científicas (CISA-INIA/CSIC), Madrid, España

*Address all correspondence to: sandrabarroso@ucm.es

IntechOpen

© 2024 The Author(s). Licensee IntechOpen. This chapter is distributed under the terms of the Creative Commons Attribution License (http://creativecommons.org/licenses/by/4.0), which permits unrestricted use, distribution, and reproduction in any medium, provided the original work is properly cited.

References

[1] World Organisation for Animal Health. African Swine Fever. Disease Card. 2021. Available from: https://www.woah.org/app/uploads/2021/03/oie-african-swine-fever-technical-disease-card.pdf [Accessed: 30 July 2024]

[2] Dixon LK, Stahl K, Jori F, Vial L, Pfeiffer DU. African swine fever epidemiology and control. Annual Review of Animal Biosciences. 2020;**8**:221-246. DOI: 10.1146/annurev-animal-021419-083741

[3] Blome S, Franzke K, Beer M. African swine fever - a review of current knowledge. Virus Research. 2020;**287**:198099. DOI: 10.1016/j.virusres.2020.198099

[4] Penrith ML, Kivaria FM, Masembe C. One hundred years of African swine fever: A tribute to R. Eustace Montgomery. Transboundary and Emerging Diseases. 2020;**67**:14183. DOI: 10.1111/tbed.14183

[5] Alonso C, Borca M, Dixon L, Revilla Y, Rodriguez F, Escribano JM, et al. ICTV virus taxonomy profile: Asfarviridae. The Journal of General Virology. 2018;**99**:613-614. DOI: 10.1099/jgv.0.001049

[6] Karger A, Pérez-Núñez D, Urquiza J, Hinojar P, Alonso C, Freitas FB, et al. An update on African swine fever virology. Viruses. 2019;**11**:864. DOI: 10.3390/v11090864

[7] Dixon LK, Stahl K, Jori F, Vial L, Pfeiffer DU. African swine fever epidemiology and control. Annual Review of Animal Biosciences. 2019;**7**:41-63. DOI: 10.1146/annurev-animal-021419-083741

[8] World Organisation for Animal Health (WOAH). World Animal Health Information Database (WAHID) Interface. 2024. Available from: https://wahis.woah.org/#/dashboards/country-or-disease-dashboard [Accessed: 30 July 2024]

[9] Government of the United Kingdom. African Swine Fever (ASF) in Asia. Available from: https://assets.publishing.service.gov.uk/media/668684564a94d44125d9ccd7/asf_asia_update_25.pdf [Accessed: 30 July 2024]

[10] Food and Agriculture Organization of the United Nations. African Swine Fever (ASF) Situation Update in Asia & Pacific. 2024. Available from: https://www.fao.org/animal-health/situation-updates/asf-in-asia-pacific/en [Accessed: 30 July 2024]

[11] Busch F, Haumont C, Penrith ML, Laddomada A, Dietze K, Globig A, et al. Evidence-based African swine fever policies: Do we address virus and host adequately? Frontiers in Veterinary Science. 2021;**8**:637487. DOI: 10.3389/fvets.2021.637487

[12] Costard S, Mur L, Lubroth J, Sanchez-Vizcaino JM, Pfeiffer DU. Epidemiology of African swine fever virus. Virus Research. 2013;**173**:191-197. DOI: 10.1016/j.virusres.2012.10.030

[13] Jori F, Bastos AD. Role of wild suids in the epidemiology of African swine fever. EcoHealth. 2009;**6**:296-310. DOI: 10.1007/s10393-009-0248-7

[14] Jori F, Vial L, Penrith ML, Perez-Sanchez R, Etter E, Albina E, et al. Review of the sylvatic cycle of African swine fever in sub-Saharan Africa and the Indian Ocean. Virus Research. 2013;**173**:212-227. DOI: 10.1016/j.virusres.2012.10.005

[15] Penrith ML, Bastos AD, Etter EM, Beltrán-Alcrudo D. Epidemiology of African swine fever in Africa today: Sylvatic cycle versus socio-economic imperatives. Transboundary and Emerging Diseases. 2019;**66**:14117. DOI: 10.1111/tbed.13117

[16] Plowright W. Vector transmission of African swine fever virus. In: Liess B, editor. Hog Cholera/Classical Swine Fever and African Swine Fever. Luxembourg: EEC Publication EUR 5904 EN; 1977. pp. 575-587

[17] Boinas FS, Wilson AJ, Hutchings GH, Martins C, Dixon LJ. The persistence of African swine fever virus in field-infected *Ornithodoros erraticus* during the ASF endemic period in Portugal. PLoS One. 2011;**6**:e20383. DOI: 10.1371/journal.pone.0020383

[18] Sanchez-Vizcaino JM, Mur L, Bastos ADS, Penrith ML. New insights into the role of ticks in African swine fever epidemiology. Revue Scientifique et Technique. 2015;**34**:503-511. DOI: 10.20506/rst.34.2.2375

[19] Niederwerder MC, Khanal P, Foland T, Constance LA, Stoian AMM, Deavours A, et al. Stability of African swine fever virus in feed during environmental storage. Transboundary and Emerging Diseases. 2022;**69**:14666. DOI: 10.1111/tbed.14666

[20] Kalmar ID, Cay AB, Tignon M. Sensitivity of African swine fever virus (ASFV) to heat, alkalinity and peroxide treatment in presence or absence of porcine plasma. Veterinary Microbiology. 2018;**219**:97-101. DOI: 10.1016/j.vetmic.2018.04.025

[21] Songkasupa T, Boonpornprasert P, Suwankitwat N, Lohlamoh W, Nuengjamnong C, Nuanualsuwan S. Thermal inactivation of African swine fever virus in feed ingredients. Scientific Reports. 2022;**12**:20290. DOI: 10.1038/s41598-022-20290-9

[22] Jurado C, Martínez-Avilés M, De La Torre A, Štukelj M, de Carvalho Ferreira HC, Cerioli M, et al. Relevant measures to prevent the spread of African swine fever in the European Union domestic pig sector. Frontiers in Veterinary Science. 2018;**5**:77. DOI: 10.3389/fvets.2018.00077

[23] Sauter-Louis C, Conraths FJ, Probst C, Blohm U, Schulz K, Sehl J, et al. African swine fever in wild boar in Europe-a review. Viruses. 2021;**13**:1717. DOI: 10.3390/v13091717

[24] Vergne T, Guinat C, Pfeiffer DU. Undetected circulation of African swine fever in wild boar, Asia. Emerging Infectious Diseases. 2020;**26**:200608. DOI: 10.3201/eid2610.200608

[25] Cadenas-Fernández E, Ito S, Aguilar-Vega C, Sánchez-Vizcaíno JM, Bosch J. The role of the wild boar spreading African swine fever virus in Asia: Another underestimated problem. Frontiers in Veterinary Science. 2022;**9**:844209. DOI: 10.3389/fvets.2022.844209

[26] Casal J, Tago D, Pineda P, Tabakovski B, Santos I, Benigno C, et al. Evaluation of the economic impact of classical and African swine fever epidemics using OutCosT, a new spreadsheet-based tool. Transboundary and Emerging Diseases. 2022;**69**:14590. DOI: 10.1111/tbed.14590

[27] Berthe F. The global economic impact of ASF. Bulletin - Office International des Épizooties. 2020;**1**:3119. DOI: 10.20506/bull.2020.1.3119

[28] Matsumoto N, Siengsanan-Lamont J, Halasa T, Young JR, Ward MP,

Douangngeun B, et al. The impact of African swine fever virus on smallholder village pig production: An outbreak investigation in Lao PDR. Transboundary and Emerging Diseases. 2021;**68**:14193. DOI: 10.1111/tbed.14193

[29] Urbano AC, Ferreira F. African swine fever control and prevention: An update on vaccine development. Emerging Microbes and Infections. 2022;**11**:2108342. DOI: 10.1080/22221751.2022.2108342

[30] World Organisation for Animal Health. African Swine Fever (Infection with African Swine Fever Virus). 2024. Available from: https://www.woah.org/fileadmin/Home/eng/Health_standards/tahm/3.09.01_ASF.pdf [Accessed: 30 July 2024]

[31] Zhang C, Li S, Zhang M, Li Y, Gimenez-Lirola LG, Li B, et al. Editorial: Diagnostics and detection of African swine fever virus. Frontiers in Veterinary Science. 2023;**10**:1195138. DOI: 10.3389/fvets.2023.1195138

[32] Bohorquez JA, Lanka S, Rosell R, Pérez-Simó M, Alberch M, Rodriguez F, et al. Efficient detection of African swine fever virus using minimal equipment through a LAMP PCR method. Frontiers in Cellular and Infection Microbiology. 2023;**13**:1114772. DOI: 10.3389/fcimb.2023.1114772

[33] Yang L, Wang L, Lv M, Sun Y, Cao J. Clinical validation of DNA extraction-free qPCR, visual LAMP, and fluorescent LAMP assays for the rapid detection of African swine fever virus. Life (Basel). 2022;**12**:1067. DOI: 10.3390/life12071067

[34] Fan X, Li L, Zhao Y, Liu Y, Liu C, Wang Q, et al. Clinical validation of two recombinase-based isothermal amplification assays (RPA/RAA) for the rapid detection of African swine fever virus. Frontiers in Microbiology. 2020;**11**:1696. DOI: 10.3389/fmicb.2020.01696

[35] Ceruti A, Kobialka RM, Ssekitoleko J, Okuni JB, Blome S, Abd El Wahed A, et al. Rapid extraction and detection of African swine fever virus DNA based on isothermal recombinase polymerase amplification assay. Viruses. 2021;**13**:1731. DOI: 10.3390/v13091731

[36] Cavalera S, Colitti B, De Mia GM, Feliziani F, Giudici SD, Angioi PP, et al. Development of molecular and antigenic-based rapid tests for the identification of African swine fever virus in different tissues. Talanta. 2023;**258**:124443. DOI: 10.1016/j.talanta.2023.124443

[37] Orosco FL. Host immune responses against African swine fever virus: Insights and challenges for vaccine development. Open Veterinary Journal. 2023;**13**:1517-1535. DOI: 10.5455/OVJ.2023.v13.i12.2

[38] Afe AE, Shen ZJ, Guo X, Zhou R, Li K. African swine fever virus interaction with host innate immune factors. Viruses. 2023;**15**:1220. DOI: 10.3390/v15061220

[39] Niu S, Guo Y, Wang X, Wang Z, Sun L, Dai H, et al. Innate immune escape and adaptive immune evasion of African swine fever virus: A review. Virology. 2023;**587**:109878. DOI: 10.1016/j.virol.2023.109878

[40] Gao Q, Yang Y, Feng Y, Quan W, Luo Y, Wang H, et al. Effects of the NF-κB signaling pathway inhibitor BAY11-7082 in the replication of ASFV. Viruses. 2022;**14**:297. DOI: 10.3390/v14020297

[41] Wu L, Yang B, Yuan X, Hong J, Peng M, Chen J, et al. Regulation and

evasion of host immune response by African swine fever virus. Frontiers in Microbiology. 2021;**12**:698001. DOI: 10.3389/fmicb.2021.698001

[42] Franzoni G, Pedrera M, Sánchez-Cordón PJ. African swine fever virus infection and cytokine response in vivo: An update. Viruses. 2023;**15**:233. DOI: 10.3390/v15010233

[43] Montoya M, Franzoni G, Pérez-Nuñez D, Revilla Y, Galindo I, Alonso C, et al. Immune responses against African swine fever virus infection. In: Understanding and Combating African Swine Fever: A European Perspective. Wageningen: Wageningen: Academic Publishers; 2021. 805-820 p. DOI: 10.3920/978-90-8686-910-7_3

[44] Nash RH. Understanding the Interactions of African Swine Fever Virus with Dendritic Cells and the Adaptive Immune Response [Doctoral Dissertation]. Surrey: University of Surrey; 2020

[45] Zhu Z, Mao R, Liu B, Liu H, Shi Z, Zhang K, et al. Single-cell profiling of African swine fever virus disease in the pig spleen reveals viral and host dynamics. Proceedings of the National Academy of Sciences of the United States of America. 2024;**121**:e2312150121. DOI: 10.1073/pnas.2312150121

[46] Bosch-Camós L, Alonso U, Esteve-Codina A, Chang CY, Martín-Mur B, et al. Cross-protection against African swine fever virus upon intranasal vaccination is associated with an adaptive-innate immune crosstalk. PLoS Pathogens. 2022;**18**:e1010931. DOI: 10.1371/journal.ppat.1010931

[47] Franzoni G, Razzuoli E, Dei Giudici S, Carta T, Galleri G, Zinellu S, et al. Comparison of macrophage responses to African swine fever viruses reveals that the NH/P68 strain is associated with enhanced sensitivity to type I IFN and cytokine responses from classically activated macrophages. Pathogens. 2020;**9**:209. DOI: 10.3390/pathogens9030209

[48] Carrasco CP, Rigden RC, Vincent IE, Balmelli C, Ceppi M, Bauhofer O, et al. Interaction of classical swine fever virus with dendritic cells. The Journal of General Virology. 2004;**85**:1633-1641. DOI: 10.1099/vir.0.19716-0

[49] Pedrera M, Soler A, Simón A, Casado N, Pérez C, Arias M, et al. Characterization of the protective cellular immune response in pigs immunized intradermally with the live attenuated African swine fever virus (ASFV) Lv17/WB/Rie1. Vaccine. 2024;**12**:443. DOI: 10.3390/vaccines12040443

[50] Sun W, Zhang H, Fan W, He L, Chen T, Zhou X, et al. Evaluation of cellular immunity with ASFV infection by swine leukocyte antigen (SLA)-peptide tetramers. Viruses. 2021;**13**:2264. DOI: 10.3390/v13112264

[51] Barroso-Arévalo S, Barasona JA, Cadenas-Fernández E, Sánchez-Vizcaíno JM. The role of interleukine-10 and interferon-γ as potential markers of the evolution of African swine fever virus infection in wild boar. Pathogens. 2021;**10**:757. DOI: 10.3390/pathogens10060757

[52] Lopez E, van Heerden J, Bosch-Camós L, Accensi F, Navas MJ, López-Monteagudo P, et al. Live attenuated African swine fever viruses as ideal tools to dissect the mechanisms involved in cross-protection. Viruses. 2020;**12**:1474. DOI: 10.3390/v12121474

[53] Zhu JJ. African swine fever vaccinology: The biological challenges

from immunological perspectives. Viruses. 2022;**2022**(14):2021. DOI: 10.3390/v14092021

[54] Muñoz-Pérez C, Jurado C, Sánchez-Vizcaíno JM. African swine fever vaccine: Turning a dream into reality. Transboundary and Emerging Diseases. 2021;**68**:2657-2668. DOI: 10.1111/tbed.14191

[55] Sang H, Miller G, Lokhandwala S, Sangewar N, Waghela SD, Bishop RP, et al. Progress toward development of effective and safe African swine fever virus vaccines. Frontiers in Veterinary Science. 2020;**7**:84. DOI: 10.3389/fvets.2020.00084

[56] Arias M, Dixon L, Gallardo C, Jori F, Laddomada A, Martins C, et al. Approaches and perspectives for development of African swine fever virus vaccines. Vaccines (Basel). 2017;**5**:35. DOI: 10.3390/vaccines5040035

[57] Shirley JL, De Jong YP, Terhorst C, Herzog RW. Immune responses to viral gene therapy vectors. Molecular Therapy. 2020;**28**:709-722. DOI: 10.1016/j.ymthe.2020.01.001

[58] Manso RJ. Déclaration sur la vaccination contre la Peste Porcine Africaine à la XXXe Session Générale de l'Office International des Epizooties. Bulletin - Office International des Épizooties. 1962;**58**:1031-1040 (In French)

[59] Petisca NJ. Quelques aspects morphologiques des suites de la vaccination contre la peste porcine Africaine (virose L) au Portugal. Bulletin - Office International des Épizooties. 1965;**63**:199-237 (In French)

[60] Sánchez-Cordón PJ, Chapman D, Jabbar T, Reis AL, Goatley L, Netherton CL, et al. Different routes and doses influence protection in pigs immunised with the naturally attenuated African swine fever virus isolate OURT88/3. Antiviral Research. 2017;**138**:1-8. DOI: 10.1016/j.antiviral.2016.11.021

[61] O'Donnell V, Holinka LG, Krug PW, Gladue DP, Carlson J, Sanford B, et al. African swine fever virus Georgia 2007 with a deletion of virulence-associated gene 9GL (B119L), when administered at low doses, leads to virus attenuation in swine and induces an effective protection against homologous challenge. Journal of Virology. 2015;**89**:8556-8566. DOI: 10.1128/JVI.00969-15

[62] Borca MV, Ramirez-Medina E, Silva E, Vuono E, Rai A, Pruitt S, et al. Development of a highly effective African swine fever virus vaccine by deletion of the I177L gene results in sterile immunity against the current epidemic Eurasia strain. Journal of Virology. 2020;**94**:e02017-e02019. DOI: 10.1128/JVI.02017-19

[63] Barasona JA, Gallardo C, Cadenas-Fernández E, Jurado C, Rivera B, Rodríguez-Bertos A, et al. First oral vaccination of Eurasian wild boar against African swine fever virus genotype II. Frontiers in Veterinary Science. 2019;**6**:137. DOI: 10.3389/fvets.2019.00137

[64] Gallardo C, Soler A, Rodze I, Nieto R, Cano-Gómez C, Fernandez-Pinero J, et al. Attenuated and non-haemadsorbing (non-HAD) genotype II African swine fever virus (ASFV) isolated in Europe, Latvia 2017. Transboundary and Emerging Diseases. 2019;**66**:1399-1404. DOI: 10.1111/tbed.13132

[65] Barasona JA, Cadenas-Fernández E, Kosowska A, Barroso-Arévalo S, Rivera B, Sánchez R, et al. Safety of African swine fever vaccine candidate

Lv17/WB/Rie1 in wild boar: Overdose and repeated doses. Frontiers in Immunology. 2021;**12**:761753. DOI: 10.3389/fimmu.2021.761753

[66] Petrini S, Righi C, Mészáros I, D'Errico F, Tamás V, Pela M, et al. The production of recombinant African swine fever virus Lv17/WB/Rie1 strains and their in vitro and in vivo characterizations. Vaccine. 2023;**11**:1860. DOI: 10.3390/vaccines11121860

[67] Wang T, Luo R, Sun Y. Current efforts towards safe and effective live attenuated vaccines against African swine fever: Challenges and prospects. Infectious Diseases of Poverty. 2021;**10**:137. DOI: 10.1186/s40249-021-00920-6

[68] Bosch-Camós L, López E, Rodriguez F. African swine fever vaccines: A promising work still in progress. Porcine Health Management. 2020;**6**:17. DOI: 10.1186/s40813-020-00154-2

Section 3

Other Conditions and Diseases

Chapter 6

Canine Genetics and Epidemiology of Behavior in Dogs

Adriana Amfim, Livia Cătălina Bercea and Natalia Cucu

Abstract

According to Acheson Roy, the constant aim in epidemiology is that of answering the question '*why did this individual develop this disease in this moment of time?*.' Similar to studies applied in classical epidemiology, observational epidemiological studies in genetics are divided into *descriptive* and *analytical*. *Descriptive* studies verify the variance model of the disease or behavior and can offer clues about the involvement of genetic or environmental factors. *Analytical* studies establish the causal effect (genetic cause) on the disease or behavior phenotype; in the case of an existing genetic cause, it remains to be identified. An analytic study model would be appropriate for the analysis of idiopathic aggressivity and epilepsy in dogs. In some cases, common etiological factors can be the basis of both situations. One such potential factor can be changes in dopaminergic function codified by the SLC6A3 gene. In the central nervous system of mammals, dopamine is a key neurotransmitter involved in locomotory activity, objectives, and reward processing-oriented behavior, as well as in convulsive activity.

Keywords: genetics, behavior, epidemiology, aggressivity, dog

1. Introduction

Behavior has a major genetic component [1, 2], and many traits are both phenotypically and genetically correlated. For example, this can happen in the case of compulsive behavior correlated with a vulnerable genetic locus in chromosome 7 in dogs [3], or with noise sensitivity correlated with distinct regions in the canine genome, which are also associated with anxiety [4].

Behavioral traits are complex, and scientifically proven to be influenced by genetic and environmental factors (e.g., maternal behavior or owner experiences) [5], and can also affect the health and well-being of dogs because personality traits are linked to mental health, especially neuroticism which was proven to predict and precede psychopathology, especially mood alterations and anxiety [6–8]. The most frequently studied personality traits in dogs are fearfulness, activity, responsiveness to training, aggression or dominance, sociability with humans and other dogs, and perseverance.

Genetic epidemiology is a novelty in veterinary medicine and proposes an exploration of the independent roles of genetic determinants and the interaction with environmental factors; it is a science that analyses interactions between the etiology, distribution, and control of diseases in related groups, and of hereditary determinism in populations. Genetic epidemiology evaluates the role of hereditary causes of diseases in families and populations, analyzes hereditary models of different particular disorders, detects and localizes genes, and uncovers markers associated with disease susceptibility by studying gene-gene or gene-environmental factor interactions. Regarding desirable or undesirable behavior manifestations, behavioral genetics aims to answer the question '*to what extent is behavior inherited?*.' Thereby, behavioral genetics attributes an important role to heredity while also evaluating aspects related to environmental factors. Epigenetics, for example, shows that prenatal exposure of a fetus to maternal stress could determine epigenetic methylation of promoter regions of the glucocorticoid receptor [9].

From an epidemiological point of view, causality analysis can also be applied in behavioral genetic studies for the evaluation of genetic factor involvement in psychobehaviors, and can help formulate answers to questions such as: '*is one intervention more efficient than another?*' or '*what are the comparative results of two alternative interventions?*' with an interventional purpose in behavior therapy. In the behavior genetics domain, the most useful epidemiological instruments used in researching risk factors can be the cohort study which allows the identification of individuals who are more at-risk than others (e.g., breed predisposition), or the case-control analysis which uncovers differences between healthy and sick individuals, analyzing the effects of many genes in association with risk factors which in a genetic context is extremely important because heredity plays a key role in genetic prophylactic programs. Epidemiological studies applied in behavioral genetics have a major role in establishing if there is a causality between exposure and pathology.

Epidemiological genetic research of dog behavior proposes going through some stages:

- Establishing a genetic component in the behavior manifestation;
- Establishing the genetic effect in relation to other variation sources that determine the risk of disease (e.g., environmental effects);
- Identification of genes responsible for the genetic component;
- Identification of the mode of hereditary transmission;
- Quantifying the risk of transmission;
- Establishing adequate measures for screening and genetic prophylaxis.

2. Genetics of dog behavior

2.1 The genetic mechanism of behavior from an epidemiological standpoint

From a *genetics* and *neurobiological* point of view, the dog can be a very good predictive study model not only for cardiac, endocrine, and oncological pathologies but also for neurological and mental illnesses in humans, which is supported by studies like the one showing a significant association between SLC6A3 40 bp-VNTR polymorphisms in dogs with idiopathic aggression and suicidal behavior in humans (aggressive manifestations and anxiety in dogs being associated with the SLC6A3 gene [10]). Other examples are the associations between ADHD in dogs and eating disorders in humans, fear and noise sensitivity in dogs that include neuropsychiatric loci in humans [4, 11], DRD4 polymorphisms in dogs that can be related to both human ADHD and canine impulsivity [12]; the apparent pathway communality in both canine and human obsessive-compulsive behavior [13], and the association between the genetic components of sociable behavior in dogs that occupy the same gene region as the social behavior in humans [14].

While the identification of genes responsible for common genetic diseases is rapidly advancing, the genes that are the basis of desirable or undesirable behaviors remain relatively unknown, necessitating interdisciplinary studies, multifactorial approaches, and complex associations through which to evaluate the associative level of a genetic etiology with a behavior pattern. For these reasons, behavioral genetics of canine psychopathology uses both genetic (genome sequencing, evaluation of genetic markers like enzymes or other proteins) and epigenetic studies (such as DNA methylation), as well as behavioral studies that use epidemiological methods of evaluation for associations and correlations. Thereby, in the last few years, there have been many studies on canine behavior, centered on the evaluation of correlations between environmental factors, breeds, and some behavioral patterns. The evaluation of genetic factor roles in the etiology of a certain behavior refers to the candidate genes through which genetic variance is examined in known loci or those suspected of playing a role in the pathogenesis of a psychopathology or that of an undesirable behavior.

The Online Mendelian Inheritance in Animals, 2024 (OMIA) database currently registers over 904 phenotypes and genetic mutations, out of which there are 607 dog genetic phenotypes that could be used as a good predictive model for genetic human pathology (e.g., hip dysplasia, Cushing disease, diabetes mellitus, diabetes insipidus, hemophilia A, XY intersexuality, or degenerative diseases such as Alzheimer's disease, or other types of nervous system diseases like epilepsy). Due to a long history of selective breeding, multiple breeds of dogs are susceptible to genetic diseases that are difficult to study in humans, such as cancer, heart disease, deafness, blindness, and autoimmune diseases. Furthermore, because they share the same environment, dogs are an important model for behavioral genetic studies in humans. Due to rigorous selection, the 'modern' dog is practically unequaled in its genetic and phenotypic diversity. More than that, each breed represents a group of phenotypically similar individuals, making them ideal for studies regarding the relationship between innate behaviors and learned behaviors, under the influence of environmental factors. Because of this, the dog is a better study model for human psychiatric disorders than rodents [15, 16].

Regarding the association between the genetic equipment and the manifestation of a certain type of behavior, there have been complex studies with both genomic sequencing and epidemiological investigation surveys, that have identified 11 unique genetic regions (or loci) of the canine genome that are strongly associated with behavior. None of these regions have specifically been associated with a certain breed, which suggests that these personality traits precede the modern selective breeding done by humans [17]. Because breed predisposition is an important factor in a lot of genetic pathologies in dogs, genetic epidemiological studies have been oriented towards exploring the relations between modern dog breeds and behavior characteristics. One major study in this field was carried out by Kathleen Morrill [18], who applied a strategy named genome-wide association study (GWAS) in order to correlate regions of the canine genome with certain traits or behavior characteristics. Data for the study was obtained from

Darwin's Ark, an open-source database with canine traits and behaviors reported by owners [18]. According to this study, behavior characteristics were influenced by many factors, including environmental and individual genetic inheritance, but a modest role was attributed to the modern breed classification. By analyzing owner-reported behavioral data for different breeds, and those of breed ancestors which were genetically detected, it was discovered that breeds have a minor contribution of only 9% to behavior manifestations. For other behavioral traits, such as directional motor models (dog's interest and interaction with toys), age was a good predictor for behavior; younger dogs had a better chance of receiving a bigger score in this category. For other traits included in the survey, such as 'leg lifting durin urination,' the dog's gender was the best behavior predictor. Physical features like coat color were five times more likely to be predicted by breed compared to behavioral traits. Thus, according to this cohort study, behavioral characteristics attributed to modern breeds are polygenic, influenced by the environment, and have a different prevalence for all breeds. Other epidemiological studies that use breed as a predictive feature of psychopathologies have shown major differences between breeds for all studied behavioral traits. One such study by Salonen et al. [19] which evaluated prevalence, comorbidities, and breed differences in anxiety in dogs, has shown that only 10.6% of miniature Schnauzers were aggressive towards strangers, compared to only 0.4% of Labrador Retrievers. In a similar manner, it was reported that 9.5% of Staffordshire Bull Terriers had manifested a tail-chasing behavior, while none of the Lagotto Romagnolo dogs had manifested this behavior [19]. An ample study realized by geneticists from the University of Helsinki collected 13,715 answers from pet owners which evaluated seven anxiety features for 264 breeds. According to this study, the dogs presented major differences in the prevalence of all anxiety-related features, suggesting a strong genetic contribution; 72.5% of dogs presented one type of disruptive behavior, the most frequent reported behavioral problems being excessive barking, destructiveness, aggression, inappropriate urinary, and fear. Approximately 20–25% of dogs manifested fear towards strangers, other dogs, or situations, and separation anxiety was noted in 14–20% of subjects; noise sensitivity was one of the most frequent anxiety features, one in three dogs manifesting excessive fear towards at least one type of sound, the reaction towards fireworks being the most frequent anxiety responses; fear being the second most frequent symptom, with a frequency of 29% [19]. Following this study's conclusions related to breeds as a predictive element, selective breeding could reduce the prevalence of anxiety in dogs.

Most epidemiological studies realized in the field of behavioral genetics have targeted undesirable behavior traits that include fear, noise sensitivity, fear of heights or certain surfaces, separation anxiety, barking, aggression towards strangers, aggression towards owners, aggression towards other dogs, hyperactivity, impulsivity, distractedness, and personality traits that include fearfulness, energy, responsiveness to training (trainability), aggression, dominance, sociability in relation to humans, sociability towards other dogs, and perseverance [16–21].

Regarding behavior phenotypes, both humans and dogs seem to develop the same characteristics in obsessive-compulsive disorder (OCD), to manifest compulsive behavior or inattention, and ADHD, aggression, or separation anxiety, in similar ways [22]. These aspects were correlated with the fact that both humans and dogs share the same environment. For a dog, the risk of developing a behavior problem can depend on a series of factors, including breed, age, sex, hormonal status (spayed, neutered, or intact), diet, relationship with owners, acquisition path, and daily time spent on specific activities. Among the epidemiological factors involved in developing a certain type of behavior, the influence of the environment on nervous system reactivity is well-known and scientifically proven, being unrelated to an individual's inherited genetic equipment. In a study on lab rats, Yamamuro et al. [23] has shown that young individuals who are socially isolated for 2 weeks after weaning, develop a series of deficiencies and defects in their prefrontal cortex, just like mice raised in conditions that favor the development of an autistic behavior, have a low risk of developing anxiety, but have a higher probability of manifesting social behavior features [23].

2.2 Epidemiological tools used in the evaluation of some behavior phenotypes or psychopathologies

Since its beginning, the field of behavioral genetics has made use of observational, descriptive, and correlational epidemiological studies, as well as longitudinal, retrospective, prospective, case-control, and prevalence studies. Regarding undesirable behaviors like aggressiveness, or neurological disorders such as idiopathic epilepsy, epidemiological investigations should establish, besides manifested phenotypes, the genetic etiology, in order to evaluate the hereditary component of these pathologies; the aim *per se* is that of limiting the transmission to descendants, because genetic determinism is a cofactor of the manifestation of a phenotype, the same hereditary component could be or not be expressed, according to environmental factor. Epidemiological studies are important for understanding the risk factors involved in behavioral problems and are subsequently the best preventive measures. Specialty literature mentions a lot of survey methods for a multifactorial evaluation of both the owner's personality, and their psychological state, as well as the training methods and behavior/temperament of the dogs, or the genetic etiology correlated with a certain behavior phenotype.

But epidemiological research into the behavioral patterns of dogs can have its limitations, thus, many transversal epidemiological studies used in behavior evaluation can be hampered by small sample sizes which limits the extrapolation of results to a specific breed, the use of a small number of features, to have an overview of the individual within a group and of individuals within a breed. This explains the observed limitations in the previously mentioned study, realized through the application of a survey-type investigation by Salonen et al. [19] in the evaluation of anxiety. Initially, only three traits were included (for approximately 3300 study participants); through the extension of the study from three to seven traits related to anxiety, they obtained four times more data for the prevalence evaluation of different behavioral problems similar to anxiety in a large population of guide dogs; comorbidity between noise sensitivity and separation anxiety has been observed, and breed-specific behavioral variance, the latter being extremely important in the evaluation of heredity in the manifestation of anxiety.

Choosing the most appropriate epidemiological investigation method is a desideratum for behavioral genetics studies, in order to avoid errors of interpretation, insufficient data, or difficult extrapolation. One suggestion that should be considered for the behavioral evaluation of dogs is that of using the *survey* as an instrument for data collection and using the *correlation* analysis method. As an example, for anxiety, the same properly mentioned study could establish different traits related to anxiety and other comorbidities, the most frequent trait being fear, especially in aggressive and hyperactive or impulsive dogs, while the second most frequent trait being noise sensitivity, especially in fearful dogs [19].

Therefore, specialized literature from the fields of epidemiology, behavioral genetics, and ethology, suggests the following epidemiological instruments in the evaluation of behaviors as being the most used:

- *The 10-item Personality Inventory (TIPI)*, a brief and validated measure of the 'big five' dimensions of human personality (owner): Agreeableness, extraversion, emotional stability, openness, and conscientiousness [24];

- *An 8-item survey* on the tendency of owners to use forceful training methods, named the Attitude to Training scale (ATT) [21];

- *'Mini' evaluation and research survey of dog behavior (mini-C-BARQ)*, a short version of the 100-item *C-BARQ*. It is a validated evaluation of canine temperament and behavior that measures 14 different behaviors, as well as a series of miscellaneous behaviors, such as creating a mess around the house and persistent barking [25];

- *Behavior phenotype studies* correlated with genetic test results through a *26-item questionnaire on the dog's behavior* [26];

- *Questionnaire with data processing through structural equation modeling (SEM)* that can be used to examine, for example, associations between metatraits like stability and biological neuroplasticity, and undesirable traits in dogs; modeling data from databases like http://darwinsark.org/ [27];

- *GWAS analysis and data correlation from behavior questionnaires* with the identification of behavior phenotypes and some loci associated with behavior traits in dogs [28];

- *Dg Personality Questionnaire (DPQ/DPQL; 45 questions)* [29];

- *Canine Health-related Quality of Life Survey (CHQLS; 11 questions)* [30];

- *Dog Impulsivity Assessment Scale (DIAS; 18 questions, including one also in DPQ)* [31];

- *Canine Cognitive Dysfunction Rating Scale (CCDR; six questions)* [32].

Standardized international protocols for testing and terminology used in behavior evaluation in dogs should be used in order to facilitate selection against behavioral disorders in the 'modern dog' and to optimize reproductive success and performance in working dogs. This review underlines common obstacles for behavioral genetics researchers and the current understanding of this topic [33].

3. A model of epidemiological approach in idiopathic aggression through psychometric evaluation instruments

Animals can manifest conspecific and heterospecific aggression in relation to resource competition (such as food and territory) and protecting descendants, while conspecific aggression can manifest in relation to competition for a mate and maintaining group hierarchy [34]. The domestic dog (*Canis lupus familiaris*), the only large carnivore that can be domesticated, can represent a significant threat to humans in aggressive interactions because aggressive behavior can appear not only in agonistic interactions (offensive-defensive) but also as predatory reactions or simply accidental clashes. Dog bites can lead to severe lesions or death and represent a major public health issue in certain countries. The evolution of aggressive behavior and its genetic and neurobiological bases present a theoretical interest in the evolution of animal behavioral trait evolution [35], and a practical importance in the context of aggression towards congenators and the interaction between people and domestic animals.

Aggressive behavior in animals manifests in a wide array of contexts, aggressiveness being the least desirable canine trait. For this reason, genetic sequencing tests are used to detect some differences in the genetic coding of neurotransmitters and their receptors in aggressive and nonaggressive dog groups in order to establish possible genetic causes. Because of research in behavioral genetics, the present-day belief is that identifying genetic polymorphisms associated with aggressive behavior no matter the breed can be useful for breeders and more so for dog owners in the context of routine genetic screening for this undesirable trait, especially for breeds considered to be high risk for manifesting aggression.

The ability to predict which individuals are predisposed towards developing an aggressive behavior that will actually manifest in time is limited, which makes for few and inefficient preventive measures. Experience has shown that some dog breeds are predisposed towards aggressive behaviors, which led to the introduction of a series of specific breed-related legislative measures, but heredity in a breed context has proven that behavior variations are insignificant; this reasoning not being scientifically proven.

The climax of half a century of canine behavior research with the help of genomic investigations, has been established by the identification of genes responsible for silver fox docility. Behavior heredity in aggressive canines was proven through the selective breeding of foxes (*Vulpes vulpes*), aggressive and tamed individuals created through selective breeding of individuals based on their response towards humans. The aggressive individuals presented differences in DNA sequences of genes involved in key pathways regulating neurologic processing, as well as different levels of specific gene expression in the brain.

Following a 50-year experiment, new genetic epidemiology studies have been reproduced through which were detected for example, a set of genes correlated with aggressive behavior through the codification of dopamine, serotonin, and glutamate receptors in some breeds like the English Cocker, or the dopamine transporter gene that is associated with impulsive behavior in the Malinois; in this way demonstrating the genetic cause of aggressive behavior in canines [36].

From a genetic point of view, the dog genome is similar in size to that of humans and other mammals, containing approximately 2.5 billion pairs of DNA bases. Although the genome acts as a model for producing morphological, physiological, and behavioral observable characteristics (meaning phenotypes), the expression of these traits is conditioned by an epidemiological variability observed in different social or ecological contexts, sometimes quantified in generations. Phenotypic variation induced by the environment which results from the expression of different genes, can be relegated by processes that do not include the DNA sequence itself, but rather epigenetic mechanisms. DNA methylation is one such epigenetic mechanism that allows organisms to respond to environmental changes through changes in gene expression and changes in phenotypes respectively. DNA methylation during early ontogenetic development can have long-term consequences on gene expression, physiology, and behavior in many vertebrates [37].

But human intervention in breeding or the perpetuation of certain defects cannot be ignored, with selective breeding or consangvinization being implemented to obtain most dog breeds, presenting a higher risk for pure-bred dogs that will have a greater risk of developing genetic disorders as a consequence of inbreeding [38]. The domestic dog is a species with a very diverse morphology, including breeds that were developed in the last few hundred years, which resulted in dramatic phenotypical variations. At present, there are 197 breeds registered with the American Kennel Club (AKC) and approximately 400 internationally recognized breeds [38], each population with its unique size, morphology, and behavioral model. Modern dog breeds have been around for less than 160 years (50–80 generations) in comparison to the origin of dogs, more than 10,000 years ago [18]; prehistoric wolves having probably adapted to using human leftovers through changes in morphology, behavior, metabolism, and breeding [39]. In contrast, modern dog breed selection for conformation to a physical ideal and descendants' purity is a Victorian invention [40], consangvinization possibly leading to a higher prevalence of recessive genetic disorders, transforming what would normally be a rare disease into a frequent one in a specific breed or family line. It can also lead to genetic load purging and elimination, associated with inbreeding depression [41].

Before the 1800s, dogs were selected primarily for functional roles such as hunting, protection, and shepherding—hereditary behaviors derived from the predatory sequence of wolves. However, studies have uncovered that behavioral variance level in a breed is close to that of variance between breeds [37] suggesting that these predictions are predisposed to errors even in pure-bred dogs. Behavioral factors show a high variability in breeds, suggesting that although the breed can influence the probability that a certain behavior will manifest, the breed alone is not, contrary to popular belief, sufficiently informative to predict a certain behavior pattern. It is believed that domestication has involved the selection for reduced agonistic aggression towards humans [42].

Even so, such a trait cannot be completely eliminated from the dog population, because it remains a vital defense mechanism, and some dogs are raised specifically for guarding and protection, where elements of agonistic manifestations are desirable. Therefore, a considerable variance can be expected in the expression of aggressive responses in some contexts between breeds [43]. Differences between dog breeds regarding behavior have been studied using a variety of instruments, including standardized tests and surveys based on questionnaires, targeting dogs, owners, instructors (trainers), and behavioral experts. Some dog breeds—mostly those historically used for guarding and dog fights—are usually considered to have more chances of developing problematic aggressive behavior, and legislation regarding the prevention of attacks on humans is usually concentrated on the restriction or interdiction of owning such a breed [44].

The Dangerous Dogs Act (1991) from Great Britain interdicts the ownership of four types of breeds, respectively Fila Brasileiro, Dogo Argentino, Japanese Tosa, and Pit Bull Terrier. A detailed hypothesis that sustains the breed-specific legislation (BSL) is the high heritability of the tendency towards aggression in dogs, with an implied existence of low variation in the breed. High heritability is necessary in order for a feature to become breed-specific or typical for a breed, as it happens with breed-related morphological features. In theory, behavioral traits typical for a breed could be reached with specific training offered to all the individuals that represent a breed, but in this case, any legislative solution should be focused on training rather than the breed itself.

High variation of a hereditary feature in a breed implies the fact that such a feature is not breed-specific; if the breed is not a good predictor of behavior in the individual, this undermines the rationality of breed-specific legislation. Aggression towards strangers has been proven to be among the behavioral components with the highest heritability between breeds (behavioral variance between breeds; h2 = 0.68) in pure-bred domestic dogs [45]; even so, a trait's heritability does not necessarily imply a low variation in breeds. A series of behavioral studies have shown a relatively high variance within breeds, in comparison to variance among breeds in a series of behavioral traits, including aggressiveness tendencies.

In consequence, a recent genomic study [45] has shown that although the majority of canine behavioral traits have a relatively high heritability (h2 > 0.25), the breed was responsible for only 9% of behavior variance between individuals. This aspect can suggest that variance in the tendency towards aggression has been maintained in breeds through generations. Alternatively, this variance can result from a relaxed selection based on behavioral traits in dog breeds, and a bigger accent on morphological features in the construction of a breed standard. Other studies [2] have discovered that behavioral answers of dogs from breeds that are monitored through legislation acts, and given a temperament test, have been classified as adequate in 95% of tested individuals and are not significantly different compared to behavior test responses in Golden Retrievers, that are generally considered to be pets without personality issues. This data could be used to argue that the legislation offers an incorrect list of breeds that present a high biting risk for humans, or that this risk is not breed-specific.

3.1 Genetic mechanism in idiopathic aggressiveness in dogs

The aggressive behavior of a dog can be caused by a poor state of health, or other elements such as the dog's upbringing and training, meaning a cumulation of exogenic factors, but also the action of endogenic hereditary factors, more specifically by the genetically inherited neurobiological pattern. Both categories of factors should be evaluated when the owner states they have '*an aggressive animal,*' '*an epileptic animal,*' or that '*their dog's behavior has changed.*' It should objectively evaluate if there are some health changes in the dog, mistakes in the dog's training, 'unknown' causes, or other factor that could determine a sudden, new, or repetitive episode.

The complete sequencing of the dog genome has provided a lot of information on the processes of evolution in canines and the genetic basis of phenotypic features in dogs and other animals. Because behavior is a consequence of the activity of the central nervous system, it is not surprising that differences in the neurobiological activity of neurotransmitters are associated with differences in behavior. Aggressiveness and idiopathic epilepsy are long-lasting problems for dog owners. In some cases, common etiological factors can be the basis for both situations. One such potential factor can be the change in the dopaminergic function of a key neurotransmitter involved in locomotor activity, objective and reward processing behaviors, and convulsive activity [46].

Serotonin is produced from tryptophane and is believed to be important in the etiology and treatment of mood disorders, including aggression in dogs [45]. Therefore, neurotransmitters or chemical mediators are chemical substances that are found in the brain and play a role in transmitting, modulating, and amplifying action potentials in synapses; knowing this, the logical conclusion is that the levels of serotonin or the number of serotonin receptors can be quantified in nonaggressive and aggressive dogs, with the prediction that serotonin levels will be lower in aggressive dogs.

Based on current studies, dopamine is the most involved neurotransmitter in aggression; studies have shown that in comparison to nonaggressive individuals, aggressive Cockers have significantly different alleles for both dopamine and serotonin receptors [45]. The gene that encodes dopamine receptors seems to also be correlated with impulsive behavior in the German Sheppard, and the dopamine transporter seems to be involved in aggression, at least in the Malinois breed.

Furthermore, the short form of the tyrosine-hydroxylase gene seems to be involved in dopamine synthesis in German Shepherd and Siberian Huskies with altered social behaviors [47]. Because of this, behavioral genetics studies on aggressive dogs aim to quantify blood and cerebrospinal fluid dopamine levels, as well as its expression in the brain. Dopamine (3-hydroxytyramine) is characterized as a neurotransmitter in both central and peripheral nervous systems. It is an organic chemical compound from the catecholamine and phenethylamine families and constitutes approximately 80% of the total catecholamines found in the brain. Dopamine (D1 and D2) is synthesized from tyrosine, catalyzed by the enzyme tyrosine kinase, has multiple receptors, and is inactivated by a different enzyme named monoaminoxidase (MAO). Although produced by less than 1% of the total neurons in the brain, dopamine mediates a variety of physiological functions and modulates behavior, being involved in the pathogenesis of a wide array of behaviors, including aggression, in part due to its neuromodulating role [48].

Dopamine is also released when dogs are waiting for a reward, in a process called *reward anticipation*, used in training, because it helps dogs reproduce past satisfying events and experiences. Too much dopamine can lead to a state of restlessness, repetitive actions (compulsive behaviors), and overexcitement. Too little dopamine can lead to lethargy, depression, social withdrawal, and lack of concentration. Therefore, there cannot be a discussion of correcting undesirable behaviors without evaluating this neurotransmitter, not only from a quantitative neurobiological standpoint but also from a genetic determinism point of view.

Regarding the genetic base of phenotypic expression, in dopaminergic modulation there is the involvement of alleles that regulate transporters, receptors, and dopamine-inactivating enzymes, this being comparable in nonaggressive versus aggressive dogs. Dopaminergic involvement in aggressive behavior is also sustained by the intervention of pharmacotherapy with dopaminergic antagonists in cases of compulsive behaviors [49]. Nevertheless, the complex polygenic nature of aggression suggests that the same genetic polymorphism combined with different environmental conditions can lead to a wide variety of behavior expressions, including presenting aggression associated with this polymorphism [50].

The dopamine transporter produced by the dopamine transporter gene (DAT) is responsible for dopamine removal from the extracellular space, as well as the regulation of action potential amplitude and duration in dopaminergic synapses. Although there is a dispute related to the probability that a DAT mutation can cause convulsions or convulsion-associated aggression, a DAT variable number tandem repetition (VNTR) in humans was involved in alcohol withdrawal symptoms. Furthermore, the higher density of dopamine striatal transporter in violent alcoholics in comparison to nonviolent alcoholics and a control group of healthy individuals sustain the involvement of the dopaminergic system in aggressive behavior. There was also a suggestion that DAT might be a common denominator in schizophrenia and epilepsy [51].

Because of these associations between the dopamine transporter, aggressive behavior, and convulsions, addressing the candidate gene is a working hypothesis for establishing the predictive value of the contribution of canine DAT in episodic aggression and convulsive activity in dogs in general, and specifically for the Malinois breed. In dogs, DAT is located on chromosome 34 (chr34:11209118-11245456), it has 18 exons and two reported transcripts. DAT is codified by the SLC6A3 gene and plays an important role in regulating the dopamine neurotransmitter.

The SLC6A3 gene contains several repeat alleles (3–11 repeats) of a 40 base pair variable number tandem repeats in the 3′-untranslated region (3′-UTR), which can influence the expression levels of DAT. Regarding the Malinois breed, a variable number of tandem repeats (VNTR) in SLC6A3 have been associated with stress-related behaviors: lowered posture, hypervigilance in different stages of training, and episodic changes in behavior which have been reported by Malinois owners in different studies in the USA [36].

Regarding breed-specific differences, idiopathic aggressivity (aggression with unknown causes) has been observed especially in Malinois dogs. Thereby, in 2013, Lit et al. [52] discovered some types of polymorphisms of a gene, identified later as SLC6A3. The first detected polymorphism was the Poly (A) insertion of 12 nucleotides highlighted mainly in the Malinois breed. This variant is associated with swift and unpredictable behavior changes. Moreover, an 18 nucleotide (Ao) deletion was also identified in most of the evaluated breeds. In the study, the authors have uncovered another variant (A10) in Boxers. Further research has proven that the SLC6A3 gene codifies a protein responsible for signal amplitude and duration in dopaminergic synapses [53] in dogs. In humans, SLC6A3 is associated with aggressiveness, hyperactivity, and reactions to novelties. Experimental research in mice for the SLC6A3 gene has uncovered significant differences between groups regarding aggressive behaviors and other social behaviors, hyper-locomotion, and the response to a new environment, which once again proves that there is a link between SLC^A3 and a series of behavioral phenotypes [54].

Due to the fact that the Malinois breed presents a particular type of idiopathic aggression (aggressiveness with unknown causes), associated with episodic convulsive seizures or with a lack of response to any type of stimuli, this rare breed has garnered a lot of attention from owners, breeders, trainers, or ethologists. In general, aggressiveness and sudden behavioral changes are associated mainly with the A22/A22 genotype. Individuals that have at least an A22 allele and have an A0/A22 or A10/A22 genotype can manifest unpredictable aggressiveness. A0/A0, A0/A10, and A10/A10 are not associated with episodic aggression (**Table 1**) [55].

Furthermore, through additional sequencing in SLC6A3, the Poly (A) intronic insertion with 12 nucleotides "PolyA (22)" before the terminal exon has been

- A0/A0 Genotype A0/A0 **is not associated** with episodic aggressiveness
- A0/A10 Genotype A0/A10 **is not associated** with episodic aggressiveness
- A10/A10 Genotype A10/A10 **is not associated** with episodic aggressiveness
- A0/A22 Genotype A0/A22 **can be associated** with an unpredictable or undesirable behavior
- A10/A22 Genotype A10/A22 **can be associated** with an unpredictable or undesirable behavior
- A22/A22 Genotype A22/A22 **is associated** with an unpredictable or undesirable behavior

Table 1.
Results of genetic testing for aggressive behavior predisposition.

associated with convulsions, "glazing over" behavior, and episodic biting behavior. Numerous epidemiologic and genetic behavioral studies have tried to classify aggressiveness phenotypes, and present-day genomic studies can answer some essential questions in the pre-and post-training behavior evaluations of some breeds.

3.2 Epidemiological evaluation of aggressiveness in the dog with an emphasis on the Malinois breed

The evolution of aggressive behavior and its genetic and neurobiological bases present a theoretical interest in the larger scope of the evolution of behavioral traits in animals, and a practical interest in the context of aggression towards humans, conspecifics, and the interaction between humans and domestic animals. Some dog breeds, mainly those historically used for specific tasks like fights and guarding, are usually considered to have a high risk of manifesting a problematic aggressive behavior. The legislation regarding the prevention of dog attacks against humans is usually focused on the restriction or interdiction o such breeds [56].

Impulsivity is an aspect of executive control which refers to the capacity of inhibiting behavior in the presence of important indices, thus the ability to control behavior using a series of cognitive processes. Specialized literature sources regarding psychiatric disorders in humans, aggressive behavior was correlated with high impulsivity and weak executive control, and in the dog, impulsivity was correlated with a high risk of aggressiveness. The dog impulsivity assessment scale (DIAS) [31] and the positive and negative activation scale (PANAS) are two validated instruments with a special relevance for the evaluation of aggression-prone behavioral tendencies. DIAS contains three factors; one of these—the Aggression Threshold and Response to Novelty—describes a specific behavior trait that can be directly relevant for the evaluation of attack risk in dogs, reflecting a relationship between the low threshold of aggression and a negative evaluation of new situations.

Sensitivity towards the affective quality of stimuli can be widely relevant for biting risk because individuals that are more aversive towards the qualities of potentially negative stimuli (beyond those associated with the uncertainty of a new situation), can be expected to become defensive. Moreover, those individuals that are sensitive to rewards can have more chances of engaging in a resource dispute, because they might have a tendency to overestimate the value or benefits of a resource. Sensitivity to rewards can be evaluated in dogs using PANAS.

In the epidemiological evaluation of idiopathic aggressiveness, both in research and in practice, a wide array of methodologies has been employed to compare dog breed behaviors, with results varying according to the method used, which makes it difficult to formulate conclusions on behavior differences between breeds. As previously stated, there have been many questionnaires developed for the evaluation of individual dogs in a large array of contexts (as opposed to the specific context of an experimental context). It has been stated that a psychometric approach that follows profiling the biological construct at the base of behavioral tendencies has the potential to offer a more consistent image of behavior tendencies compared to arbitrary traits or behavior experiments [48].

It also allows for a fast collection of data from a large number of individuals, which is extremely important when comparing behavior traits between groups with large variances within the group. However, depending on the design, some psychometric questionnaires offer just one instrument for individual behavior difference evaluation, without identifying traits that are significant either on a psychological level or a functional biological one. Constructing a more complex questionnaire involves formulating more elements in order to avoid inexact answers which are either intentional or resulting from not understanding the questions. Another approach, apart from the complex questionnaire, could be the multidisciplinary approach to aggression correlated with anxiety in dogs, for example, according to the human model proposed by the latest research carried out in Romania. Using the classic instruments from psychology, for measuring stress (DASS-21R, QOLI, CD questionnaires), and correlating the obtained molecular results, it was possible to compare the psychoemotional area with the molecular one, thus achieving an additional criterion of more subtle differentiation in terms of changes at the molecular (epigenetic) level. Thus, the psychoemotional correlation for the assessment of stress, anxiety, and depression in humans with somatic stress can highlight the diagnostic potential of some epigenetic markers (miR-21 and miR-26) with a role in preventive medicine [57].

No.	Genotype SLC6A3—Poly (A22) for genetic predisposition to aggression	Behavior phenotype	Answer—evaluation questionnaire for genetic predisposition to aggression
1.	**Heterozygote N/A22**	a. Convulsions b. **Glassy eyes** c. Aggressiveness (without factors)	a. No b. **Yes** c. No
2.	**Homozygote N/N**	a. Convulsions b. Glassy eyes c. **Aggressiveness (without factors)**	a. No b. No c. **Yes**
3.	Homozygote N/N	a. Convulsions b. Glassy eyes c. Aggressiveness (without factors)	a. No b. No c. No
4.	Homozygote A22/A22	a. Convulsions b. Glassy eyes c. Aggressiveness (without factors)	a. No b. No c. No
5.	**Heterozygote N/A22**	a. **Convulsions** b. **Glassy eyes** c. **Aggressiveness (without factors)**	a. **Yes** b. **Yes** c. **Yes**
6.	**Heterozygote N/A22**	a. Convulsions b. Glassy eyes c. Aggressiveness (without factors)	a. No b. No c. No

Phenotypes manifestations of behavior directly related with predisposition to aggression in Malinois breed on SLC6A3 polymorphism gene.

Table 2.
Associations between the PolyA (22) allele and behavioral phenotypes.

The *dichotomous questionnaire* contains of set of data for dog identification, habitat, health status, medical and behavior history. This questionnaire is inspired by the DBQ (Dog Behavior Questionnaire), the latter being one of the SAB Test questionnaires (Socially Acceptable Behavior). Owner answers receive dichotomous codification (**Yes, No**) for any affirmative response to questions regarding changes in dog behavior. The SAB Test was initially created for the evaluation of aggressive behavior in dogs in the Netherlands but is successfully used in evaluating aggressiveness and temperament in many other countries. This trast contains more subtests and questionnaires, including DBQ.

Regarding the evaluation of idiopathic aggressiveness with genetic determinism especially in the Malinois breed, this can be achieved through correlation studies between genetic testing results and gene expression throughout the generation of a behavior phenotype, in order to identify a predictive behavior associated with the specific genetic polymorphism, with the aim of understanding some behavior phenotypes related to SLC6A3 (**Table 2**). The dichotomous questionnaire can show if there are associations between the PolyA (22) allele and behavioral changes in dogs, according to owner reporting, if the aggressive behavior is associated with a medical pathology, a lack of exercise or a poor state of health. Moreover, the questionnaire can be successfully used in correlation with a genetic test, and in the determination of the perfect metho of sport training for the Belgian Malinois. It is worth mentioning that the analysis of any behavior remains somewhat subjective and cannot be truly quantified, making it almost impossible to define and accurately measure behaviors through questionnaires, due to the fact that owner opinions could be subjective.

4. Conclusions

Genetic epidemiology represents a novelty in the veterinary medical field and evaluates, both in the context of family and that of the population, the role of hereditary causes of diseases; it analyzes hereditary models; it detects and localizes genes, and uncovers markers associated with disease susceptibility, by studying.

Canine behavioral psychopathology with a genetic substrate uses both genetic (genome sequencing, evaluation of genetic markers like enzymes or other proteins) or epigenetic (such as DNA methylation) studies, as well as behavioral studies that employ epidemiologic evaluation methodss of association or correlation relationships (e.g., dog impulsivity assessment scale—DIAS).

It seems that aggressive behavior is dominated by polygenic features, inherited and expressed differently according to environmental factors and individual complex expressions.

In conclusion, we can say that dog behavior is defined not only by the genetic selection through which genotypes with the desired phenotypical expression are obtained, but also by housing conditions, growth and development, training, neonatal experiences, maternal behavior, and all related factors.

Conflict of interest

The authors declare no conflict of interest.

Notes/thanks/other declarations

Thanks to my daughter, Ioana Teodora Amfim, for the documentation.

Appendices and nomenclature

GWAS	genome-wide association study
SLC6A3 40 bp-VNTR	40 bp variable number tandem repeat (VNTR) in SLC6A3
ADHD	attention deficit hyperactivity disorder
OCD	obsessive-compulsive disorder
AKC	American kennel club
BSL	breed-specific legislation
DAT	dopamine transporter gene

Author details

Adriana Amfim[1,2]*, Livia Cătălina Bercea[1] and Natalia Cucu[2,3,4]

1 Faculty of Veterinary Medicine, Spiru Haret University, Bucharest, Romania

2 Association for Epigenetics and Metabolomics, Bucharest, Romania

3 Faculty of Biology, Genetics Department, University of Bucharest, Bucharest, Romania

4 "Constantin Angelescu" Interdisciplinary Advanced Research Institute, Bucharest, Romania

*Address all correspondence to: adriana.amfim@gmail.com

IntechOpen

© 2024 The Author(s). Licensee IntechOpen. This chapter is distributed under the terms of the Creative Commons Attribution License (http://creativecommons.org/licenses/by/4.0), which permits unrestricted use, distribution, and reproduction in any medium, provided the original work is properly cited.

References

[1] Ilska J, Haskell MJ, Blott SC, Sánchez-Molano E, Polgar Z, Lofgren SE, et al. Genetic characterization of dog personality traits. Genetics. 2017;**206**(2):1101-1111. DOI: 10.1534/genetics.116.192674

[2] Hradecká L, Bartoš L, Svobodová I, Sales J. Heritability of behavioural traits in domestic dogs: A meta-analysis. Applied Animal Behaviour Science. 2015;**170**:1-13. DOI: 10.1038/s41398-018-0361-x

[3] Dodman NH, Karlsson EK, Moon-Fanelli A, Galdzicka M, Perloski M, Shuster L, et al. A canine chromosome 7 locus confers compulsive disorder susceptibility. Molecular Psychiatry. 2009;**15**(1):8-10. DOI: 10.1038/mp.2009.111

[4] Sarviaho R, Hakosalo O, Tiira K, Sulkama S, Salmela E, Hytönen MK, et al. Two novel genomic regions associated with fearfulness in dogs overlap human neuropsychiatric loci. Translational Psychiatry. 2019;**9**:18. DOI: 10.1038/s41398-018-0361-x

[5] Tiira K, Hakosalo O, Kareinen L, Thomas A, Hielm-Björkman A, Escriou C, et al. Environmental effects on compulsive tail chasing in dogs. PLoS One. 2012;**7**(7):e41684. DOI: 10.1371/journal.pone.0041684

[6] Widiger TA. Introduction. In: Widiger TA, editor. The Oxford Handbook of the Five Factor Model. Oxford, UK: Oxford Library of Psychology; 2017. pp. 1-8. DOI: 10.1093/oxfordhb/9780199352487.013.9

[7] Hengartner MP, Kawohl W, Haker H, Rössler W, Ajdacic-Gross V. Big Five personality traits may inform public health policy and preventive medicine: Evidence from a cross-sectional and a prospective longitudinal epidemiologic study in a Swiss community. Journal of Psychosomatic Research. 2016;**84**:44-51. DOI: 10.1016/j.jpsychores.2016.03.012

[8] Kotov R, Gamez W, Schmidt F, Watson D. Linking "big" personality traits to anxiety, depressive, and substance use disorders: A meta-analysis. Psychological Bulletin. 2010;**136**(5):768-821. DOI: 10.1037/a0020327

[9] Overall LK, Tiira K, Broach D, Bryant D. Genetics and behavior: A guide for practitioners. Veterinary Clinics of North America: Small Animal Practice. 2014;**44**(3):483-505. DOI: 10.1016/j.cvsm.2014.01.006

[10] Piotti P, Satchell LP, Lockhart TS. Impulsivity and behaviour problems in dogs: A reinforcement sensitivity theory perspective. Behavioural Processes. 2018;**151**:104-110. DOI: 10.1016/j.beproc.2018.03.012

[11] Zmorzyński S, Styk W, Klinkosz W, Iskra J, Filip AA. Personality traits and polymorphisms of genes coding neurotransmitter receptors or transporters: Review of single gene and genome-wide association studies. Annals of General Psychiatry. 2021;**20**(1):7. DOI: 10.1186/s12991-021-00328-4

[12] Bonvicini C, Cortese S, Maj C, Baune BT, Faraone SV, Scassellati C. DRD4 48 bp multiallelic variants as age-population-specific biomarkers in attention-deficit/hyperactivity disorder. Translational Psychiatry. 2020;**10**(1):70. DOI: 10.1038/s41398-020-0755-4

[13] Noh HJ, Tang R, Flannick J, O'Dushlaine C, Swofford R,

Howrigan D, et al. Integrating evolutionary and regulatory information with a multispecies approach implicates genes and pathways in obsessive-compulsive disorder. Nature Communications. 2017;**8**(1):774. DOI: 10.1038/s41467-017-00831-x

[14] Persson ME, Wright D, Roth LS, Batakis P, Jensen P. Genomic regions associated with interspecies communication in dogs contain genes related to human social disorders. Scientific Reports. 2016;**29**(6):33439. DOI: 10.1038/srep33439

[15] Overall KL. Natural animal models of human psychiatric conditions: Assessment of mechanism and validity. Progress in Neuropsychopharmacology and Biological Psychiatry. 2000;**24**(5):727-776. DOI: 10.1016/s0278-5846(00)00104-4

[16] Salonen M, Mikkola S, Hakanen E, Sulkama S, Puurunen J, Lohi H. Personality traits associate with behavioral problems in pet dogs. Translational Psychiatry. 2022;**12**:78. DOI: 10.1038/s41398-022-01841-0

[17] Dog genetics suggest that behavior is more than just breed [Internet]. Available from: https://www.broadinstitute.org/news/dog-genetics-suggest-behavior-more-just-breed [Accessed: June 21, 2024]

[18] Morrill K, Hekman J, Li X, McClure J, Logan B, Goodman L, et al. Ancestry-inclusive dog genomics challenges popular breed stereotypes. Science. 2022;**376**(6592):eabk0639. DOI: 10.1126/science.abk0639

[19] Salonen M, Sulkama S, Mikkola S, Puurunen J, Hakanen E, Tiira K, et al. Prevalence, comorbidity, and breed differences in canine anxiety in 13,700 Finnish pet dogs. Scientific Reports. 2020;**10**(1):2962. DOI: 10.1038/s41598-020-59837-z

[20] Martínez G, Pernas GS, Casalta FJD, Suárez Rey ML, De la Cruz LFP. Risk factors associated with behavioral problems in dogs. Journal of Veterinary Behavior. 2011;**6**(4):225-231. DOI: 10.1016/j.jveb.2011.01.006

[21] Dodman NH, Brown DC, Serpell JA. Associations between owner personality and psychological status and the prevalence of canine behavior problems. PLoS One. 2018;**13**(2):e0192846. DOI: 10.1371/journal.pone.0192846

[22] Vas J, Topál J, Péch E, Miklósi A. Measuring attention deficit and activity in dogs: A new application and validation of a human ADHD questionnaire. Applied Animal Behaviour Science. 2007;**103**(1-2):105-117. DOI: 10.1016/j.applanim.2006.03.017

[23] Yamamuro K, Bicks LK, Leventhal MB, Kato D, Im S, Flanigan ME, et al. A prefrontal-paraventricular thalamus circuit requires juvenile social experience to regulate adult sociability in mice. Nature Neuroscience. 2020;**23**(10):1240-1252. DOI: 10.1038/s41593-020-0695-6

[24] Gosling DS, Rentfrow PJ. Swann WB.A very brief measure of the big-five personality domains. Journal of Research in Personality. 2003; **37**(6):504-528. DOI: 10.1016/S0092-6566(03)00046-1

[25] Wilkins V, Evans J, Park C, Dog Aging Project Consortium, Fitzpatrick AL, Creevy KE, et al. Validation of the shortened version of the canine behavioral assessment and research questionnaire (C-BARQ) using participants from the dog aging project. PLoS One. 2024;**19**(4):e0299973. DOI: 10.1371/journal.pone.0299973

[26] Takeuchi Y, Kaneko F, Hashizume C, Masuda K, Ogata N, Maki T, et al. Association analysis between canine behavioural traits and genetic polymorphisms in the Shiba Inu breed. Animal Genetics. 2009;**40**(5):616-622. DOI: 10.1111/j.1365-2052.2009.01888.x

[27] Salonen M. Complex traits, complex results: the genetic, demographic, and environmental factors of cat and dog behavior [thesis]. Faculty of Veterinary Medicine: University of Helsinki, Folkhälsan Research Center; 2020

[28] Li JH, Mazur CA, Berisa T, Pickrell JK. Low-pass sequencing increases the power of GWAS and decreases measurement error of polygenic risk scores compared to genotyping arrays. Genome Research. 2021;**31**(4):529-537. DOI: 10.1101/gr.266486.120

[29] Jones AC. Development and validation of a dog personality questionnaire [thesis]. The University of Texas at Austin ProQuest Dissertations & Theses; 2008

[30] Lavan RP. Development and validation of a survey for quality of life assessment by owners of healthy dogs. The Veterinary Journal. 2013;**197**(3):578-582. DOI: 10.1016/j.tvjl.2013.03.021

[31] Wright HF, Mills DS, Pollux PMJ. Development and validation of a psychometric tool for assessing impulsivity in the domestic dog (*Canis familiaris*). International Journal of Comparative Psychology. 2011;**24**(2):210-225. DOI: 10.46867/ijcp.2011.24.02.03

[32] Salvin HE, McGreevy PD, Sachdev PS, Valenzuela MJ. The canine cognitive dysfunction rating scale (CCDR): A data-driven and ecologically relevant assessment tool. The Veterinary Journal. 2011;**188**(3):331-336. DOI: 10.1016/j.tvjl.2010.05.014

[33] van Rooy D, Arnott ER, Early JB, McGreevy P, Wade CM. Holding back the genes: Limitations of research into canine behavioural genetics. Canine Genetics Epidemiology. 2014;**10**(1):7. DOI: 10.1186/2052-6687-1-7

[34] Creedon N, Ó'Súilleabháin PS. Dog bite injuries to humans and the use of breed-specific legislation: A comparison of bites from legislated and non-legislated dog breeds. Irish Veterinary Journal. 2017;**21**(70):23. DOI: 10.1186/s13620-017-0101-1

[35] Tritsch NX, Sabatini BL. Dopaminergic modulation of synaptic transmission in cortex and striatum. Neuron. 2012;**76**(1):33-50. DOI: 10.1016/j.neuron.2012.09.023

[36] Lit L, Belanger JM, Boehm D, Lybarger N, Haverbeke A, Diederich C, et al. Characterization of a dopamine transporter polymorphism and behavior in Belgian Malinois. BMC Genetics. 2013;**14**:45. DOI: 10.1186/1471-2156-14-45

[37] Mehrkam LR, Wynne C. Behavioral differences among breeds of domestic dogs (*Canis lupus familiaris*): Current status of the science. Applied Animal Behaviour Science. 2014;**155**:12-27. DOI: 10.1016/j.applanim.2014.03.005

[38] Reisen J. The most popular dog breeds of 2020 [Internet]. Available from: https://www.akc.org/expert-advice/dog-breeds/the-most-popular-dog-breeds-of-2020/ [Accessed: May 30, 2024]

[39] Lord K, Feinstein M, Smith B, Coppinger R. Variation in reproductive traits of members of the genus Canis with special attention to the domestic dog (Canis familiaris). Behavioural Processes. 2013;**92**:131-142. DOI: 10.1016/j.beproc.2012.10.009

[40] Worboys M, Strange JM, Pemberton N. The invention of the modern dog: Breed and blood in Victorian Britain. The American Historical Review. 2021;**126**(2):855-856. DOI: 10.1093/ahr/rhab231

[41] Wellmann R, Pfeiffer I. Pedigree analysis for conservation of genetic diversity and purging. Genetics Research (Camb). 2009;**91**(3):209-219. DOI: 10.1017/S0016672309000202

[42] Hare B, Tomasello M. Human-like social skills in dogs? Trends in Cognitive Sciences. 2005;**9**:439-444. DOI: 10.1016/j.tics.2005.07.003

[43] Peiman KS, Robinson BW. Ecology and evolution of resource-related heterospecific aggression. The Quarterly Review of Biology. 2010;**85**(2):133-158. DOI: 10.1086/652374

[44] Allcock T, Campbell ML. The UK Dangerous Dogs Act: Improved, but legally and ethically flawed. Veterinary Record. 2021;**189**(3):e24. DOI: 10.1002/vetr.24

[45] MacLean EL, Snyder-Mackler N, vonHoldt BM, Serpell JA. Highly heritable and functionally relevant breed differences in dog behaviour. Proceedings Biological Science. 2019;**286**(1912):20190716. DOI: 10.1098/rspb.2019.0716

[46] Wilson AJ, Gelin U, Perron MC, Réale D. Indirect genetic effects and the evolution of aggression in a vertebrate system. Proceedings Biological Science. 2009;**276**(1656):533-541. DOI: 10.1098/rspb.2008.1193

[47] Amat M, Manteca X, Mariotti VM, Ruiz de la Torre JL, Fatjó J. Aggressive behavior in the English cocker spaniel. Journal of Veterinary Behavior. 2009;**4**(3):111-117. DOI: 10.1016/j.jveb.2008.08.010

[48] Sheppard G, Mills D. The development of a psychometric scale for the evaluation of the emotional predispositions of pet dogs. International Journal of Comparative Psychology. 2002;**15**:2. DOI: 10.46867/C4G30W

[49] Patel BD, Barzman DH. Pharmacology and pharmacogenetics of pediatric ADHD with associated aggression: A review. Psychiatric Quarterly. 2013;**84**(4):407-415. DOI: 10.1007/s11126-013-9253-7

[50] Gonçalves VF, Tiwari AK, de Luca V, Kong SL, Zai C, Tampakeras M, et al. DRD4 VNTR polymorphism and age at onset of severe mental illnesses. Neuroscience Letters. 2012;**519**(1):9-13. DOI: 10.1016/j.neulet.2012.04.027

[51] Le Strat Y, Ramoz N, Pickering P, Burger V, Boni C, Aubin HJ, et al. The 3′ part of the dopamine transporter gene DAT1/SLC6A3 is associated with withdrawal seizures in patients with alcohol dependence. Alcoholism: Clinical and Experimental Research. 2008;**32**(1):27-35. DOI: 10.1111/j.1530-0277.2007.00552.x

[52] Lit L, Belanger JM, Boehm D, Lybarger N, Oberbauer AM. Differences in behavior and activity associated with a poly(a) expansion in the dopamine transporter in Belgian Malinois. PLoS One. 2013;**8**:12. DOI: 10.1371/journal.pone.0082948

[53] Mortensen OV, Amara SG. Dynamic regulation of the dopamine transporter. European Journal of Pharmacology. 2003;**479**(1-3):159-170. DOI: 10.1016/j.ejphar.2003.08.066

[54] Perona MT, Waters S, Hall FS, Sora I, Lesch KP, Murphy DL, et al. Animal models of depression in dopamine, serotonin, and norepinephrine transporter knockout mice: Prominent

effects of dopamine transporter deletions. Behavioural Pharmacology. 2008;**19**(5-6):566-574. DOI: 10.1097/FBP.0b013e32830cd80f

[55] Lit L, Belanger JM, Boehm D, Lybarger N, Oberbauer AM. Dopamine transporter single nucleotide polymorphisms (SNPs) in Belgian Malinois dogs. Animal Genetics. 2013;**44**(5):604-605. DOI: 10.1111/age.12040. Epub 2013 Apr 9

[56] Hammond A, Rowland T, Mills DS, Pilot M. Comparison of behavioural tendencies between "dangerous dogs" and other domestic dog breeds - evolutionary context and practical implications. Evolutionary Applications. 2022;**19**(15-11):1806-1819. DOI: 10.1111/eva.13479

[57] Pătac B, Zăgrean A-M, Botezatu A, Fudulu A, Cucu N, Popa-Velea O, et al. The impact of health & wellness coaching intervention on the level of stress perceived physically/mentally/psychologically. Health, Sport & Rehabilitation Medicine. 2024;**25**(2): 70-79. DOI: 10.26659/pm3.2024.25.2.70

Chapter 7

Major Infertility Problems of Crossbred Dairy Cattle in Debre Berhan Milk Shed Areas

Tewodros Eshete, Tilaye Demisse, Tefera Yilma and Berhan Tamir

Abstract

The present study was conducted to determine the occurrences and features of repeat breeding and postpartum anestrous in crossbred dairy cattle. A longitudinal prospective study was carried out on 371 pregnant dairy cows to determine the occurrences of repeat breeding and postpartum anestrus. Ultrasonographic examination was undertaken on repeat breeder and postpartum anestrus cows to identify the features of repeat breeding and postpartum anestrus in crossbred dairy cows. The incidence of postpartum anestrous and repeat breeding in crossbred dairy cattle was high at 40.9 and 38.2%, respectively. From cows or heifers recorded as repeat breeders, 59.2% of cows and heifers had regular estrous cycle and functional corpus luteum, while the remaining 40.8% of dairy cows had no regular estrous cycle and functional corpus luteum in ultrasonographic examination of utero-ovarian conditions. From the cows recorded as postpartum anestrus, 34.7% of cows were true anestrus, 54.7% of cows were subestrus, and the remaining 10.5% of cows were with cystic ovary. The present study indicated that 22.6% of total dairy cows examined under the present study could not conceive within 1 year of postpartum due to repeat breeding syndrome. Moreover, 40.8% of repeat breeder dairy cows were conceived after a repeated number of services within 1 year of postpartum.

Keywords: crossbred dairy cattle, infertility, postpartum anestrous, repeat breeding, reproductive disorders, risk factors

1. Introduction

Reproductive disorders are the most severe problems affecting dairy cows' production, reproductive performance, and profitability of dairy farms in Ethiopia [1, 2]. The most common and significant reproductive problems of dairy cattle are anestrus, repeat breeding, abortion, dystocia, retained fetal membrane (RFM), endometritis, and prolapse (uterine and vaginal), all of which have a direct impact on reproductive performance and efficiency [3–5].

Though repeat breeding and postpartum anestrus are two of the most severe reproductive problems affecting dairy cattle breeding in Ethiopia [6], resulting in significant economic losses for dairy producers due to additional inseminations, increased days open and calving intervals, decreased reproductive and productive performances, and higher culling rates of potentially valuable cows. Repeat breeding, with a high incidence resulting in dairy cow infertility and significant economic loss in the dairy industry [7, 8].

A repeat breeder dairy cattle is typically defined as a sub-fertile cow or heifer that has been served three or more times with a fertile bull or inseminated with fertile sperm but fails to conceive and repeatedly returns to estrus in the absence of any apparent pathological disorder in the genital tract [7, 9, 10]. Repeat breeding is the most common yet poorly understood problem affecting dairy cattle reproduction rate, calf crop, and milk production economy [11]. Repeat breeding syndrome is an expensive impediment to effective dairy production because it causes the age of first calving in heifers to be delayed and the inter-calving interval to be lengthened, lowering the calf crop [12]. In several studies, the prevalence of repeat breeding in Ethiopia ranged from 1.3 to 28% [3, 13], with a high incidence of 61.7% also reported in crossbred dairy cattle [14].

The causes of repeat breeding were often shown to be very complex, but they can be summarized as follows: (1) management factors: bad timing of inseminations, failure to detect heat, and unprofessional insemination; (2) semen factors: low quality of semen or infertile bull; (3) cow factors: uterine infection, ovulatory defect, follicular cyst, adhesions, antibodies to seminal antigen, inappropriate uterine involution, infectious diseases, and anovulatory heats; (4) environmental factors: heat stress, nutritional factor [15–17]. Moreover, repeat breeders frequently have delayed ovulation and a prolonged follicular phase, which promotes follicle development but delays the luteinizing hormone (LH) surge, which results in relatively old follicles and oocytes by the time of ovulation [18].

Postpartum anestrus is a state of complete sexual inactivity with no manifestation of estrus for more than 2 months after calving [19], with no growing follicles becoming mature enough to ovulate [20]. Postpartum anestrus constitutes about 2/3rd of the infertility problems in crossbred dairy cows [21], and this is the most prevalent reproductive problem in dairy cows [22, 23] with calving interval to increase significantly [24–27].

Also, 40% of cows that resume cyclicity in high-producing dairy farms are not detected in estrus even when they complete one or more ovarian cycles [25]. Environmental factors like heat stress, poor nutrition, and barn conditions potentially prolong the postpartum anestrus [28]. Roelofs et al. [26] concluded that long postpartum anestrus, poor estrus detection, and poor pregnancy rates contributed to extending the calving interval of dairy cows. The long duration of postpartum anestrus negatively influences dairy cows' reproductive performance and efficiency [25].

However, in Ethiopia, studies on reproductive problems in dairy cattle are few and mainly concentrate on urban and peri-urban areas, despite these conditions being the subject of extensive research worldwide [29]. Information from the present study, which focused on identifying the occurrences of repeat breeding and postpartum anestrus and their associated risk factors, has not yet been well documented to indicate the extent of occurrences of repeat breeding and postpartum anestrus in crossbred dairy cattle. Therefore, the present study was conducted to determine the occurrences of repeat breeding and postpartum anestrus in crossbred dairy cows and to identify risk factors associated with the occurrences of repeat breeding and postpartum anestrus in Debre Berhan milk shade.

2. Material and methods

2.1 Study areas

This study was conducted in the Debre Berhan milk shed area (Debre Berhan metropolitan city), north Shoa zone, Ethiopia. The area is situated 130 km northeast of Addis Ababa. It was located between longitude 39°29′ and 39°44′ east and at a latitude 9°34′ and 9°54′2″ north with an elevation range from 2056 to 3744 m.a.s.l [30]. The mean minimum and maximum monthly temperature of the study area ranges from 2.8 to 21.9°C and the mean minimum and maximum annual rainfall ranges from 698.5 to 1083.5 mm [31].

2.2 Study animals

A total of 371 (186 for repeat breeding and 185 for postpartum anestrus) crossbred pregnant and lactating cows from 24 smallholder farms (purposively selected at approximately 35% the total population with parities zero to five parities and age 2 to 8 years old were used for this study. Cows were raised with smallholder dairy farms in intensive production systems. All herds were housed in a barn with concrete floor and corrugated iron roof. Pregnant cows and heifers were separated into maternity pens. All animals fed feedstuffs consisted of grass hay, wheat straw, barley straw, brewery byproduct, and concentrate mixture (wheat bran, wheat middling, noug seed cake, and salt). All animals were fed a mixture of brewery byproduct and roughage feed (barley straw, wheat straw, and hay) as a basal diet. Concentrate supplement was restricted to calves, milking cows, and pregnant cows (mainly during the third trimester of pregnancy).

2.3 Study design

A longitudinal study design was used to estimate incidence and characterize repeat breeding and postpartum anestrus in crossbred dairy cattle. A total of 371 pregnant crossbred dairy cows were continuously followed for the occurrences of repeat breeding and postpartum anestrus. A repeat breeder was defined as a dairy cow that did not become pregnant after three inseminations, despite no clinically detectable reproductive disorders [8]. Otherwise, dairy cow conceived within three inseminations were considered to have normal fertility [32].

In addition, all reproductive performance data such as days in milk at first AI (DIM) at first AI, first AI conception rate, number of days from calving to conception, and number of services per conception were collected. Dairy cows that were not detected in estrous for more than 60 days postpartum were examined by transrectal ultrasonography to identify and characterize postpartum anestrous. The findings were categorized as follows: (a) cows having inactive ovaries (have no CL and follicles) and without any abnormality in the uterus were categorized as true postpartum anestrus; (b) cows having active ovaries with functional CL on at least one of the ovaries were categorized as subestrus [27].

Data on the following parameters were carefully recorded on a cow basis (age, parity, milk production, and BCS) and on herd basis (frequency of anestrus and repeat breeding cows).

2.4 Statistical analysis

Data on from the record and observational study were coded and entered into a Microsoft Excel spreadsheet. The data were analyzed using SPSS software version 25. Data from repeat breeder and normal fertility cow days in milk at first AI, calving to conception interval, and number of services per conception were analyzed using one-way ANOVA. The incidence rate was used as the measure of occurrences of postpartum anestrus and repeat breeding per 100 dairy cows recruited in the study. The chi-square ($\chi 2$) statistic was used to determine the associations between predictor variables and incidence of repeat breeding and postpartum anestrus.

3. Results and discussion

3.1 Incidence and features of repeat breeding in crossbred dairy cattle

The present study revealed that 38.2% (71/186) of cows and/or heifers were repeat breeders served more than three times but not conceived (4.9 ± 1.01 NS) (**Table 1**). Of the cows reported to be repeat breeders (n = 71), 59.2% (42/71) had regular estrus cycle and functional CL, and 40.8% (29/71) had no regular estrus cycle and functional CL but had growing follicles. In the ultrasonographic examination of utero-ovarian conditions, cows or heifers reported to be repeat breeders during a longitudinal prospective study.

3.2 Reproductive performance of crossbred dairy cows

The number of dairy cows conceived within 1 year of postpartum was 77.4%, this indicated that 22.6% of dairy cows could not conceive due to repeat breeding syndrome. Days in milk at first AI, first AI conception rate, calving to conception interval, and number of services per conception were 75.9 ± 21.7, 8.7%, 215.6 ± 85.6, and 3.4 ± 0.7 d, respectively (**Table 2**). Only 40.8% of repeat breeder dairy cows were conceived after a repeated number of services within 1 year of postpartum, which was significantly ($P < 0.05$) lower than the conception rate (100%) of normal fertility dairy cows within 1 year of postpartum. The result indicated that the remaining 59.2% of repeat breeder dairy cows were not conceived, this is a huge economic loss for the dairy industry in the study areas. The number of services per conception in repeat breeder dairy cow/heifers was significantly higher compared to normal fertility dairy cows.

Descriptors	Dairy cattle examined (N)	Dairy cattle affected (N)	Incidence (%)
Normal fertility cows	186	115	61.8
Repeat breeder	186	71	38.2
RB cows had regular estrus cycle & CL	71	42	59.2
RB cows had Irregular estrus cycle & no CL	71	29	40.8

RB, means repeat breeder, N, means number, Cl, means Corpus lutiem.

Table 1.
Occurrences and features of repeat breeding in crossbred dairy cattle.

Descriptors	Normal fertility cows	Repeat breeder cows	P value
Number of Cows	115	71	—
Days in milk at first AI	76.7 ± 23.6 d	70.6 ± 43.8 d	>0.05
FAICR (%)	(8.7)	0	<0.05
Cows conceived ≤1 year postpartum (%)	100	40.8	<0.05
CCI (days)	119.8 ± 38.4	247.2 ± 97.6	<0.05
NSPC	2.3 ± 0.7	4.9 ± 1.01	<0.05
Total cows conceived within 1 year		77.4%	

FAICR, means first Artificial insemination conception rate, CCI, means calving to conception interval, and NSPC, means number of services per conception.

Table 2.
Reproductive performances of crossbred dairy cows in the study area.

Descriptors	No. cows examined	No. of cows affected	Incidence (%)
Cyclic cows (not anestrus)	185	110	59.5
Postpartum anestrus	185	75	40.5
Subestrus	75	41	54.7
True anestrus	75	26	34.7
Anestrus cows with cystic ovary	75	8	10.6

Table 3.
Occurrences and features of postpartum anestrus in crossbred cows.

3.3 Occurrences and features of postpartum anestrus in crossbred cows

The present study revealed that 40.5% (75/185) of cows were postpartum anestrus at more than 60 days postpartum. From the cows recorded as postpartum anestrus (n = 75), 34.7% (26/75) were true postpartum anestrus evidenced by having inactive ovary and no functional CL, and 54.7% (41/75) subestrus (silent heat/ovulation postpartum anestrus) defined by the presence of CL on at least one ovary in the ultrasonographic examination. Of the remaining eight postpartum anestrus cows 10.6% (8/75) were diagnosed with cystic ovary (**Table 3**).

4. Discussion

The occurrences of repeat breeding in dairy cows or heifers were wide-ranging in different environmental conditions, management conditions, and breeds [8, 33]. In the present study, the occurrence of repeat breeding was relatively high, reaching an average of 38.2%, compared to several studies on the occurrences of repeat breeding in different parts of Ethiopia [2, 14, 34, 35]. The present study fairly agrees with previous reports from different parts of the world [36, 37].

The causes of this high occurrence of repeat breeding in the present study were yet to continue, unclear, and it is multifactorial. Katagiri and Takahashi [7] stated that the causes of infertility in repeat breeder cows are vague but probably mentioned environmental, management conditions, and animal factors. Moreover, repeat-breeder cows are subject to the same problems of fertilization failure and embryonic mortality [7]. The occurrences of repeat breeding in dairy cows have increased due to inadequate estrous detection, resulting in errors in timing of insemination concerning the onset of standing estrous, or insemination of cows not in estrous [8]. Poor quality of semen and insemination techniques [38, 39], cervical or uterine infection [40], endocrine disorders, and early embryonic death [41, 42] were mentioned as the potential causes of repeat breeding in dairy cows.

Reproductive performances of crossbred dairy cows involved in the present study, like days in milk at first AI and number of services per conception, have seemed comparable to previous studies [8, 32, 43]. In line with the present study, Yusuf et al. [32] reported the first AI conception rate was much lower, and the calving to conception interval showed much longer. This was probably caused by inadequate nutrition and poor health care of dairy cows, resulting in a lower first AI conception rate and longer calving to conception interval. Cows under poor management conditions, including inadequate nutrition and cows exposed to external environment heat or cold stress had lower oocyte quality [44], reduced duration and intensity of estrous, altered follicular development, and impaired embryonic development [45], a higher incidence of abnormal resumption of postpartum ovarian cycles, a lower heat detection rate, a lower first AI conception rate, and a lower pregnancy rate [46].

In the present study, the higher (40.5%) occurrence of postpartum anestrus was found in crossbred dairy cows. This is comparable with previous research findings in Ethiopia [47, 48], while a higher prevalence of 61.7 and 49% were reported by Kibre et al. [14] and Haile et al. [29], respectively. The current study also discovered that not all postpartum anestrus cows had the same characteristics. A higher proportion of postpartum anestrus cows were subestrus, which means that they had silent estrus/silent ovulation, and a lower proportion of postpartum anestrus cows were true anestrus, which had inactive ovaries and no corpus lutetium. Yusuf et al. [32] strongly support this finding. Therefore, subestrus is more likely to occur because of inadequate estrus detection and a high incidence of silent estrus/ovulation [24, 49] and inaccurate estrus detection is one of the major problems of dairy cow [24, 50]. The most crucial management factor influencing anestrus in postpartum cows is estrous detection [51], which also determines the length of time before insemination [52] and preserves a short calving interval. Furthermore, a major contributing factor to the occurrence of postpartum anestrus is also ovarian dysfunction, which includes delayed postpartum ovarian activity and stopping cyclical ovarian activity after a period of normal ovarian function [28, 53]. The first postpartum ovulation date in cows is partially determined by their energy status, with a high incidence of postpartum anestrus that is primarily aggravated by underfeeding and poor BCS [28]. Cows with poor and excessive or fat body condition were more likely to be true anestrus at more than 60 days postpartum [8].

Furthermore, a drop in BCS indicates negative energy balance (NEB) because the cow has mobilized body fat to meet the energy demand for milk production during early lactation, which is closely associated with reproductive efficiency [54]. Poor nutrition is the primary cause of poor body condition, which leads to infertility in dairy cattle [54, 55]. The other contributing factors for high occurrences of postpartum anestrus and repeat breeding in dairy cows were high milk yield in early lactation and poor management situation [54]. Poorly maintained dairy cows are more likely to experience a negative energy balance, which impairs the release of reproductive hormones and increases the risk of fertilization failure or early embryonic death, both of which raise RB [56].

High milk yield changes in reproductive physiology [25] and an increase in the number of services per conception, higher milk supply capacity has been associated with lower fertility in dairy cows [57], leading to lower fertility rates [58].

Previous studies [59, 60] indicated that there is a clear correlation among BCS, plasma hormones (leptin, insulin, and IGF-L), LH, and initiation of ovarian activity at the postpartum period. In the study area and elsewhere in Ethiopia, the large majority of dairy farmers do not provide proper nutrition during transition and the early postpartum period. Due to that, similar to the present study, the occurrence of postpartum anestrus is high in Ethiopia [47, 48]. In cows with undernutrition reduces LH pulse frequency [61] and plasma hormones, including leptin, which can enhance pituitary LH secretion and facilitate ovarian activity in postpartum cows.

The higher incidence of postpartum anestrus due to older age and pluriparous cows is most likely because of repeated exposure of the older and pluripara genital tract to environmental factors, resulting in uterine infections and uterine involution being significantly delayed as parity and age increased, and the time between calving and ovarian resumption being also extended [35]. Moreover, older cows, especially those who gave birth to too many calves, were exposed to repeated traumatic damage of the reproductive tract and, hence, have poorly regenerating endometrium [61, 62].

5. Conclusion

The current study revealed that high occurrences of repeat breeding and postpartum anestrus in crossbred dairy cattle reduced reproductive performances and fertility in dairy cows. Poor estrus detection is a more serious problem than true anestrus, as evidenced by the higher proportion of subestrus among cows diagnosed with anestrus. Based on review of previous studies poor BCS, high milk yield, old age, high number of parity, and poor management conditions of dairy cattle were predominant factors contributing to the high incidence of postpartum anestrus and repeat breeding in dairy cattle. Dairy cattle producers should be aware and be recommended to improve feeding, housing, and health care management of dairy cattle to reduce exposure to the occurrence of repeat breeding and postpartum anestrus. To reduce RB and postpartum anestrus, dairy producers should be trained on proper handling cows in late gestation, at calving, and early postpartum periods.

Acknowledgements

The authors thank Addis Ababa University Research and Technology Transfer and thematic research "optimizing dairy herd structure and performance by increasing dairy replacement heifers, application of selected assisted reproductive techniques, and sexed sperm for funding on hormones used and data on collection." It gives me great pleasure to express my gratitude to the North Shoa Livestock Production and Promotion office and the dairy farms' owners, managers, and employees for their real collaboration and provision of the necessary information during the research period.

Conflict of interest

The authors declare that they have no conflict of interest.

Author details

Tewodros Eshete[1*], Tilaye Demisse[2], Tefera Yilma[2] and Berhan Tamir[3]

1 Department of Animal Science, College of Agriculture and Natural Resource Science, Debre Berhan University, Debre Berhan, Ethiopia

2 Department of Veterinary Obstetrics and Gynecology, College of Veterinary Medicine and Agriculture, Addis Ababa University, Bishoftu, Ethiopia

3 Department of Animal Production Studies, College of Veterinary Medicine and Agriculture, Addis Ababa University, Bishoftu, Ethiopia

*Address all correspondence to: tedyshet@gmail.com

IntechOpen

© 2024 The Author(s). Licensee IntechOpen. This chapter is distributed under the terms of the Creative Commons Attribution License (http://creativecommons.org/licenses/by/4.0), which permits unrestricted use, distribution, and reproduction in any medium, provided the original work is properly cited.

References

[1] Gizaw M, Bekana M, Abayneh T. Major reproductive health problems in smallholder dairy production in and around Nazareth town, Central Ethiopia. International Journal on Veterinary Medicine. 2007;**2**:78-81

[2] Hunduma D. The major reproductive disorders of dairy cows in and around Asella town, Central Ethiopia. Journal of Veterinary Medicine and Animal Health. 2013;**5**:113-117

[3] Gashaw A, Worku F, Mulugeta S. Assessment of smallholder dairy production system and their reproductive health veterinary medicine international problems in Jimma town, Southwest Ethiopia. International Journal of Applied Research. 2011;**9**(1):80-86

[4] Tesfaye D, Shamble A. Reproductive health problems of cows under different management systems in Kombolcha, Northeast Ethiopia. Advances in Biology Research. 2013;**7**(3):104-108

[5] Benti D, Zewdie W. Major reproductive health problems of indigenous Borena cows in Ethiopia. Journal of Advanced Veterinary and Animal Research. 2014;**1**(4):182-188

[6] Hebert AB, Bouchard E, Dutremblay D, Lefebure R. Effects of reproductive disorder and parity on repeat breeder status and culling of dairy cows. Canadian Journal of Veterinary Research. 2011;**75**(2):147-151

[7] Katagiri S, Takahashi Y. Changes in EGF concentrations during estrous cycle in bovine endometrium and their alterations in repeat breeder cows. Theriogenology. 2004;**62**:103-112. DOI: 10.1016/j.theriogenology.2003.08.019

[8] Yusuf M, Nakao T, Ranasinghe RMSBK, Gautam G, Long ST, Yoshida C, et al. Reproductive performance of repeat breeders in dairy herds. Theriogenology. 2010a;**73**:1220-1229

[9] Purohit GN. Recent developments in the diagnosis and therapy of repeat breeding cows and buffaloes. CAB Reviews: Perspectives in Agriculture, Veterinary Science, Nutrition and Natural Resources. 2008;**3**(62):1-33

[10] Asaduzzaman KM, Bhuiyan MMU, Rahman MM, Bhattacharjee J. Prevalence of repeat breeding and its effective treatment in cows in selected areas of Bangladesh. Journal of Veterinary Medicine. 2016;**14**(2):183-190

[11] Khair A, Alam MM, Rahman AKMA, Islam MT, Azim A, Chowdhury EH. Incidence of reproductive and productive diseases of crossbred dairy cattle in Bangladish. Bangladish Journal of Veterinary Medicine. 2013;**11**(1):31-36

[12] Thakur S, Singh M, Vasishta NK. Study on etiology of repeat breeding in Himanchal Pradesh. Punjab Veterinary Journal. 2006;**4**:27-29

[13] Gebrekidan B, Yilma T, Solmon F. Major causes of the slaughter of female cattle in Addis Ababa Abattoir enterprise, Ethiopia. Indian Journal of Animal Research. 2009;**43**:271-274

[14] Kibre D, Ashebir G, Gebrekidan B, Fesseha H. Study on factors affecting estrus synchronization in smallholder dairy farming systems of Tigray, northern Ethiopia. Veterinary Medicine International. 2022

[15] Spicer LJ. Proteolytic degradation of insulin-like growth factor binding

proteins by ovarian follicles: A control mechanism for selection of dominant follicles. Biology of Reproduction. 2004;**70**:1223-1230

[16] Ferreira RM, Ayres H, Chiaratti MR, Ferraz ML, Araújo AB, Rodrigues CA, et al. The low fertility of repeat-breeder cows during summer heat stress is related to a low oocyte competence to develop into blastocysts. Journal of Dairy Science. 2011;**94**(5):2383-2392

[17] Cenariu J, Josep E. Management of repeat breeding syndrome in cows. Bulletin UASVM Veterinary Medicine. 2017;**74**(2):102-107. DOI: 10.15835/buasvmcn-vm:0045. Print ISSN 1843-5270; Electronic ISSN 1843-5378

[18] Noakes DE. Arthur's Veterinary Reproduction and Obstetrics EBook. Elsevier Health Sciences; 2009

[19] Takele A, Gizaw Y, Bekana M. Major reproductive health problems in holder dairy production in and around Nazreth town, Central Ethiopia [DVM thesis]. Debrezeiet, Ethiopia: Faculty of Veterinary Medicine, Addis Ababa University; 2005

[20] Montiel F, Ahuja C. Body condition and suckling as factors influencing the duration of postpartum anestrus in cattle: A review. Animal Reproduction Science. 2005;**85**(1-2):1-26

[21] Kutty CI, Ramachandran K. Bovine infertility A field-oriented categorization based on investigation among crossbred cattle in a district of Kerala. Indian Journal of Animal Science. 2003;**73**(2):35-37

[22] Chaudhari CF, Suthar BN, Sharma VK, Dabas VS, Chaudhari NF, Panchasara HH. Estrus induction and fertility response in delayed pubertal Kankrej heifers treated with Norgestomet ear implant. Veterinary World. 2012;**5**:453-458

[23] Savalia KK, Dhami AJ, Hadiya KK, Patel KR. Augmenting fertility of anoestrus and repeat breeding buffaloes using controlled breeding techniques under field conditions. Indian Veterinary Journal. 2014a;**89**:23-27

[24] Shamsuddin M, Bhuiyan MMU, Chanda PK, Alam MGS, Galloway D. Radioimmunoassay of milk progesterone as a tool for fertility control in smallholder dairy farms. Tropical Animal Health and Production. 2006;**38**:85-92

[25] Lucy MC. Fertility in high-producing dairy cows: Reasons for the decline and corrective strategies for sustainable improvement. Society of Reproduction Fertility and Supplementation. 2007;**64**:237-254

[26] Roelofs J, López Gatius F, Hunterd RHF, van Eerdenburge FJCM, Hanzenf C. Review: When is a cow in estrous clinical and practical aspects. Theriogenology. 2010;**74**:327-344

[27] Kamal MM, Rahman MM, Momont H, Shamsuddin M. Underlying disorders of postpartum anoestrus and effectiveness of their treatments in crossbred dairy cows. Asian Journal of Animal Science. 2012;**6**:132-139

[28] Opsomer G, Grohn YT, Hertl J, Coryn M, Deluyker H, de Kruif A. Risk factors for postpartum ovarian dysfunction in high producing dairy cows in Belgium: A field study. Theriogenology. 2000;**53**:841-857

[29] Haile A, Tsegaye Y, Tesfaye N. Assessment of major reproductive disorders of dairy cattle in urban and per urban area of hosanna, southern Ethiopia. Animal Veterinary Science. 2014;**2**(5):135-141

[30] Yohannes H, Soromessa T, Argaw M, Dewan A. Changes in landscape composition and conjuration in the Beressa watershed, Blue Nile basin of Ethiopian highlands: Historical and future exploration. Heliyon. 2020;**6**:28-35. Available from: https://creativecommons.org/licenses/by-nc-nd/4.0/

[31] Ema (Ethiopia Meteorology Agency). Weather Data of North Shoa Zone from Debre Berhan and Debre Berhan Station from 1986 to 2017. Ethiopia: Ethiopia Meteorology Agency; 2017

[32] Yusuf M, Rahim L, Asja MA, Wahyudi A. The incidence of repeat breeding in dairy cows under tropical conditions. Media Peternakan. 2012;**1**(66):28-31

[33] Ayana G, Gudeta T. Incidence of major clinical reproductive health problems of dairy cows at Bako livestock research farm over two years. Animal and Veterinary Sciences. 2015;**3**(6):158-165

[34] Makonnen AB, Tadesse G, Khar SK, Bitsue HK. Efficacy of a modified Gnrh-PGF2 combination for Estrous synchronization in dairy cattle. Global Veterinary. 2016;**16**(2):200-205

[35] Esheti G, Moges N. Major reproductive health disorders in crossbred dairy cows in Ada'a district, east Shoa, Ethiopia. Global Veterinary. 2014;**13**(4):444-449

[36] Perez-Marin CC, Espana F. Oestrus expression and ovarian function in repeat breeder cows, monitored by ultrasonography and progesterone assay. Reproduction Domesticated Animal. 2007;**42**:449-456

[37] Gustafsson H. Characterisation of the repeat breeding syndrome in Swedish dairy cattle. Acta Veterinary Science and Research. 2002;**43**:115-125

[38] Hallap T, Nagy S, Jaakma Ü, Johannisson A, Rodriguez-Martinez H. Usefulness of a triple fluorochrome combination Merocyanine 540/Yo-Pro 1/Hoechst 33342 in assessing membrane stability of viable frozen-thawed spermatozoa from Estonian Holstein AI bulls. Theriogenology. 2006;**65**:1122-1136

[39] Morrell J. Update on semen technologies for animal breeding. Reproduction in Domestic Animals. 2006;**41**:63-67

[40] Moss N, Lean I, Reid J, Hodgson DR. Risk factors for repeat-breeder syndrome in New South Wales dairy cows. Preventive Veterinary Medicine. 2002;**54**(2):91-103

[41] Bage R, Gustafsson H, Larsson B, Forsberg M, RodríguezMartínez H. Repeat breeding in dairy heifers: Follicular dynamics and estrous cycle characteristics concerning sexual hormone patterns. Theriogenology. 2002;**57**:2257-2269

[42] Lopez-Gatius F, Yaniz JL, Santolaria P. Reproductive performance of lactating dairy cows treated with cloprostenol at the time of insemination. Theriogenology. 2004;**62**:677-689

[43] Santos JEP, Thatcher WW, Chebel RC, Cerri RLA, Galvão KN. The effect of embryonic death rates in cattle on the efficacy of estrus synchronization programs. Animal Reproduction Science. 2004;**82**:513-535

[44] Leroy JL, Van Soom A, Opsomer G, Goovaerts IGF, Bols PEJ. Reduced fertility in high-yielding dairy cows: Are the oocyte and embryo in danger? Part II. Mechanisms linking nutrition and reduced oocyte and embryo quality in high-yielding dairy cows. Reproduction in Domestic Animals. 2008;**43**:623-632

[45] Jordan ER. Effects of heat stress on reproduction. Journal of Dairy Science. 2003;**86**(E. Suppl.):E104-E114

[46] Kornmatitsuk B, Chantaraprateep P, Kornmatitsuk S, Kindahl H. Different types of postpartum luteal activity affected by the exposure of heat stress and subsequent reproductive performance in Holstein lactating cows. Reproduction in Domestic Animals. 2008;**43**:515-519

[47] Shiferaw Y, Tenhagen BA, Bekana M, Kassa T. Reproductive disorders of crossbred dairy cows in the central highlands of Ethiopia and their effect on reproductive performance. Tropical Animal Health and Production. 2005;**37**(5):427-441

[48] Nishi SA, Sarder MJ, Islam MH, Josim UM, Sharmin S. Management factors influencing Anestrus problems in dairy cows. Journal of Vaccines and Vaccination. 2018;**9**(3):1-4

[49] Lyimo ZC, Nkya R, Schoonman L, Van Eerdenburg FJCM. Postpartum reproductive performance of crossbred dairy cattle on smallholder farms in sub-humid coastal Tanzania. Tropical Animal Health Production. 2004;**36**:269-279

[50] Shamsuddin M. Fertility trend and status of estrus detection in the bovine under farm conditions in Bangladesh. Bangladesh Veterinary Journal. 1995;**29**:9-16

[51] Van Vliet JH, Van Eerdenburg FJCM. Sexual activities and oestrous detection in lactating Holstein cows. Applied Animal Behaviour Science. 1996;**50**:57-69

[52] Lyimo ZC, Nielen M, Ouweltjes W. Relationship among estradiol, cortisol and intensity of estrous behaviour in dairy cattle. Teriogenology. 2000;**53**:1783-1795

[53] Matiko MK, Kanuya NL, Waldmann A, Ropstad E, Reksen O. Environmental constraints on postpartum ovarian activity in Tanzanian Zebu cows. Teriogenology. 2008;**69**: 896-904

[54] Ciptadi G, Nasich M, Budiarto Nuryadi A, Nurgiartiningsih VM. The Estrus synchronization response following PGF2α treatment in Indonesian Madura cattle with different body condition scores. Journal of Animal and Veterinary Advances. 2012;**11**:676-680

[55] Schroeder UJ, Staufenbiel R. Methods to determine body fat reserves in the dairy cow with special regard to ultrasonographic measurement of backfat thickness. Journal of Dairy Science. 2006;**89**(1):1-14. DOI: 10.3168/jdsS0022-0302(06)72064-1

[56] Butler WR. Nutritional interactions with reproductive performance in dairy cattle. Animal Reproduction Science. 2000;**60**:449-457

[57] Robert SJ. Veterinary Obstetrics and Genital Diseases. 3rd ed. Dublin, Ireland: Theriogenology, Edwards' Brothers, Inc; 2011

[58] Wiltbank MC, Sartori R, Herlihy MM, Vasconcelos JLM, Nascimento AB, Souza AH, et al. Managing the dominant follicle in lactating dairy cows. Theriogenology. 2011;**76**:1568-1582

[59] León HV, Hernández-Cerón J, Keislert DH, Gutiérrez CG. Plasma concentrations of leptin, insulin-like growth factor-I, and insulin in relation to changes in body condition score in heifers. Journal of Animal Science. 2004;**82**(445):451

[60] Hess BW, Lake SL, Scholljegerdes EJ, Weston TR, Nayigihugu V, Molle JDC,

et al. Nutritional controls of beef cow reproduction. Journal of Animal Science. 2005;**83**:E90-E106

[61] Zieba DA, Amstalden M, Williams GL. Regulatory roles of leptin in reproduction and metabolism a comparative review. Domesticated Animal Endocrinol. 2005;**29**:166-185

[62] Ball P, Peters A. Reproduction in Cattle. 3rd ed. Australia: Blackwell; 2004. p. 216

Chapter 8

The Evolving Menace: Emerging *Escherichia* Species and Their Implications for Animals and Public Health

Afagh Torkan and Mahdi Askari Badouei

Abstract

While the bacterium *Escherichia coli* is a well-known member of the human gut microbiota, newer members of the genus *Escherichia* are increasingly being recognized as emerging public health threats. These species have been isolated from various animal hosts, including livestock, pets, and wildlife, as well as from human clinical samples. The genus *Escherichia* has been expanded as novel species such as *E. fergusonii*, *E. albertii*, *E. marmotae*, *E. ruysiae*, and *E. whittamii* have been added. Concerning reports have linked these *Escherichia* newcomers to a variety of severe illnesses, such as hemolytic uremic syndrome (HUS), diarrhea, and systemic infections in humans and animals. Their apparent ability to cause disease in a wide range of hosts raises worrying questions about their zoonotic potential and ability to cross species barriers. As these *Escherichia* species continue to be identified more frequently, further focus is needed to understand their epidemiology and public health implications to develop effective prevention and control strategies. Currently, the scientific community is actively working to stay ahead of these evolving *Escherichia* threats through improved detection, prevention, and control strategies to protect both animals and humans.

Keywords: emerging *Escherichia*, *E. fergusonii*, *E. albertii*, *E. marmotae*, *E. Ruysiae*, *E. Whittamii*, public health, antimicrobial resistance

1. Introduction

The genus *Escherichia* encompasses a diverse group of bacteria that are of great importance in both human and animal health. While the most well-known member of this genus is *Escherichia coli*, recent years have seen the discovery and characterization of several newly described *Escherichia* species, including *Escherichia marmotae*, *Escherichia ruysiae*, and *Escherichia whittamii* [1–3]. While the widely known *Escherichia coli* has been the primary subject of extensive investigation, the emergence and increasing recognition of novel *Escherichia* species have recently garnered significant attention [4–6].

The growing awareness of these emerging *Escherichia* species is of paramount importance, as they are believed to have the potential to impact both animal and public health. *Escherichia fergusonii*, for instance, has been associated with various infections in humans, including bacteremia, inflammatory bowel disease, wound infection, hemolytic uremic syndrome, cystitis, urinary tract infections, osteomyelitis, uveitis, and biliary infection [7–17]. Similarly, *Escherichia albertii* has been mostly linked to gastroenteritis and diarrheal illnesses and outbreaks in humans. Importantly, both *E. fergosonii* and *E. albertii* have been isolated from a variety of symptomatic and asymptomatic animal sources, raising concerns about its zoonotic potential [6, 18–21].

The diverse ecological niches occupied by these novel *Escherichia* strains, ranging from environmental sources to animal reservoirs, further heighten the concerns about their potential impact on public health and veterinary medicine. Their unique virulence factors and adaptive capabilities may confer enhanced pathogenicity, necessitating improved diagnostic and surveillance measures [4]. Moreover, the possibility of novel disease transmission pathways involving these emerging species underscores the need for a comprehensive understanding of their taxonomy, genetics, and biology.

Antimicrobial resistance is a growing concern among the novel *Escherichia* species. *Escherichia fergusonii*, for example, has been reported to exhibit resistance to various antibiotics, including ampicillin, trimethoprim-sulfamethoxazole, ceftriaxone, tetracycline, and a wide range of other antimicrobials [22–25]. Recent studies highlighted the emergence of plasmid-mediated colistin resistance (*mcr-1* gene) in *Escherichia fergusonii*, compromising the effectiveness of last-resort antibiotics [26, 27]. This resistance is particularly worrisome, as these antibiotics are commonly used in the treatment of *Escherichia*-related infections in severe infections. *Escherichia albertii*, on the other hand, has been found to harbor resistance genes for beta-lactams, tetracyclines, and sulfonamides, further complicating the management of infections caused by this species [28–30]. The emergence of multidrug-resistant strains among these novel *Escherichia* species underscores the urgent need for enhanced diagnostic capability, antimicrobial stewardship, and the development of new therapeutic options. These findings underscore the need for continued surveillance and research on AMR in *Escherichia* species, including the newly described taxa, to inform effective control and prevention strategies.

The diagnosis and pathogenesis of these novel *Escherichia* species can be complex. *Escherichia fergusonii* and *E. albertii*, for instance, can be challenging to distinguish from other *Escherichia* species using traditional biochemical tests, necessitating the use of more advanced molecular techniques for accurate identification [31–34]. *Escherichia albertii*, on the other hand, has been associated with the production of Shiga toxin, a potent virulence factor that can contribute to the development of severe diarrheal illnesses and therefore might be misreported as Shiga toxin-producing *E. coli* (STEC); furthermore, some strains exhibit Intimin, an outer membrane attachment protein encoded by *eae* gene and therefore can be misreported as enteropathogenic *E. coli* (EPEC) [35–38]. Understanding the unique pathogenic mechanisms employed by these emerging *Escherichia* species is crucial for the development of effective diagnostic tools and targeted treatment strategies.

The prevalence and distribution of novel *Escherichia* species in both domestic animal populations and human communities have been the subject of increasing attention. The presence of these emerging species in diverse animal reservoirs raises concerns about its potential for cross-species transmission and zoonotic infections [4, 5, 39].

This chapter will provide a comprehensive overview of the current state of knowledge regarding these novel *Escherichia* species, exploring their taxonomy, genetics and antimicrobial resistance profiles as well as their implications for animal and public health. By examining the latest research and highlighting the potential threats posed by these emerging strains, this chapter aims to inform and guide future scientific investigations, risk assessment, and public health strategies. By understanding the broader context of this important bacterial genus, we can better address the public health challenges posed by *Escherichia* in clinical and environmental settings.

2. Historical aspects, *Escherichia* taxonomy and nomenclature

The genus *Escherichia* has a rich and complex taxonomic history, reflecting the continual advancement in our understanding of this diverse group of bacteria. First described by Theodor Escherich in 1885 as *Bacterium coli commune* from the fecal material of neonates, the bacterium was subsequently renamed *Escherichia coli* and comprised a single species within the genus *Escherichia* [4]. Over the subsequent decades, several additional *Escherichia* species have been identified and characterized, each contributing to the evolving taxonomy of this important bacterial genus.

From the mid-twentieth century, further diversification within the *Escherichia* genus has occurred, with the discovery of novel species to the genus [4, 40]. These species, while closely related to *E. coli*, demonstrating distinct phenotypic and genotypic characteristics, underscoring the need for a more comprehensive understanding of *Escherichia* taxonomy. It is believed that the accurate identification of novel species is difficult using phenotypic characteristics but the advent of several molecular methods improved the reliable identification of novel emerging species in recent years [4, 33, 34].

In the twenty-first century, the advent of advanced molecular techniques and genome sequencing has led to the identification of other novel *Escherichia* species, further expanding the boundaries of this genus. *Escherichia marmotae*, isolated from the feces of a woodchuck (*Marmota himalayana*), that was first described in 2015 [41]. Similarly, *Escherichia ruysiae* and *Escherichia whittamii* were proposed as new species in 2016 and 2021, respectively, based on their distinct phylogenetic and genomic characteristics [2, 3].

To provide a comprehensive overview of the *Escherichia* genus, **Table 1** summarizes the known species, and their first descriptions, and **Table 2** provides taxonomic changes or reclassifications that have occurred over time. The table also highlights the phylogenetic relationships between the species, organized into broader taxonomic clades.

The discovery of novel *Escherichia* species, such as *E. albertii*, *E. fergusonii*, *E. marmotae*, and *E. whittamii*, has expanded the known diversity within the genus and challenged the traditional taxonomic boundaries [2, 3, 40, 41, 46, 51]. These findings have prompted continuous revisions to the taxonomy and nomenclature of the *Escherichia* genus, as new isolates and genomic data have become available. Because of the complex diversity and the resulting taxonomic challenges, it has been proposed that *Escherichia spp.* may be better described as species-complex [4]. It should be noted that few species previously classified as *Escherichia* species has been re-classified to other genus as summarized in **Table 2**.

The ongoing discovery and characterization of novel *Escherichia* species, as demonstrated by the examples above, highlight the dynamic nature of this genus and the continued efforts to refine its taxonomy. Understanding the historical context and the

Species	First description	Taxonomic changes	Phylogenetic groups/cryptic clades
Escherichia coli	Escherich, 1885, Migula 1895, Castellani and Chalmers 1919 [4, 42]	Originally named *Bacterium coli commune*, reclassified to *Escherichia coli* in 1919	Core *Escherichia*: A, B, C, D, E, F, G, and several E. Clades [43–45]
Escherichia fergusonii	Farmer et al. [46]	Proposed as a novel *Escherichia* species	Clade I, II [44, 47]
Escherichia albertii	Huys et al. [40]	Proposed as a novel *Escherichia* species, previously misidentified as *E. coli*/ *Hafnia*-like	Clade I, II [6]
Escherichia marmotae	Liu et al. [41]	Proposed as a novel *Escherichia* species, isolated from *Himalayan marmot* feces	Clade V [47]
Escherichia ruysiae	van der Putten et al. [3]	Proposed as a novel *Escherichia* species	Clades III and IV [47]
Escherichia whittamii	Gilroy et al. [2, 48]	Proposed as a novel *Escherichia* species	Clade II [2]

Table 1.
Historical timeline, nomenclature and phylogeny of Escherichia *species.*

Former name (*Escherichia* genus)	Current name after re-classification	References
Escherichia hermannii	*Atlantibacter hermanii*	Brenner [49] Hata [50]
Escherichia vulneris	*Pseudoescherichia vulneris*	Brenner [51] Alnajar and Gupta [52]
Escherichia blattae	*Shimwella blattae*	Burgess [53] Preist and Barker [54]
Escherichia adecarboxylata	*Leclercia adecarboxylata*	Tamura [55]

Table 2.
Former species belonging to the genus Escherichia *that are currently re-classified to other genera.*

evolving classification of *Escherichia* species is crucial for researchers and clinicians to stay abreast of the latest developments in this field, which has important implications for animal and public health.

3. Phylogenetic structure of *Escherichia* species

Comprehensive phylogenetic analyses, incorporating whole-genome sequencing data, have provided a more nuanced understanding of the relationships among the various *Escherichia* species and phylogroups. These studies have revealed complex evolutionary trajectories, with evidence of horizontal gene transfer, niche adaptation, and the emergence of novel lineages, all of which contribute to the remarkable diversity observed within this genus [43, 56].

The *Escherichia* genus is composed of several distinct phylogenetic lineages that have been classified into various phylogroups. The well-studied of these is the *Escherichia* coli phylogroups, which encompasses the majority of strains associated with human and animal infections. Within *E. coli*, seven main phylogroups (A, B1, B2, C, D, E, and F) have been described based on core genome multilocus sequence typing data [43, 56]. Interestingly, a new phylogroup, designated as phylogroup G, has recently been described that phylogenetically lies between B1 and F phylogroups. This phylogroup is distinct from the previously known *E. coli* phylogroups and exhibits a high degree of genetic diversity, encompassing both commensal and pathogenic strains [45]. The identification of phylogroup G highlights the ongoing evolution and diversification within the *Escherichia* genus.

In addition to the *E. coli* phylogroups, several cryptic *Escherichia* clades have been identified, which are genetically distinct from *E. coli* but are closely related [44, 57]. As presented in **Table 1** most novel and emerging *Escherichia* species has been classified within these cryptic clades so far. These cryptic clades, often referred to as *Escherichia* clades I-V, represent distinct evolutionary lineages within the genus and have been shown to exhibit varying degrees of host specificity and pathogenic potential [47, 58].

It should be noted that the emerging and novel *Escherichia* species, such as *E. albertii*, *E. fergusonii*, *E. marmotae*, *E. ruysiae*, and *E. whittamii*, are also closely related to *E. coli* phylogroups but have been classified as separate species based on genomic and phenotypic differences [47, 58].

Recent comparative genomic studies have revealed that *E. albertii*, *E. fergusonii*, and the cryptic *Escherichia* clades exhibit significant genetic divergence from the core *E. coli* phylogroups [41, 43, 58]. These emerging *Escherichia* species likely represent distinct evolutionary lineages that have adapted to diverse environmental niches and host associations. Further research is needed to fully elucidate the phylogenetic structure, ecological roles, and potential public health implications of these novel *Escherichia* taxa. The phylogenetic relationships and taxonomic boundaries between these newly delineated *Escherichia* species are still under investigation.

4. Epidemiology of *Escherichia* species in domestic animals

4.1 *Escherichia fergusonii*

The genus *Escherichia* encompasses a diverse group of bacteria, with several emerging species beyond the well-known *Escherichia coli*. One such species, *Escherichia fergusonii*, has gained increasing attention due to its potential implications for animal and public health and its association with various disease conditions in livestock or wildlife. *Escherichia fergusonii* has been reported in a wide range of domestic and wild animal species, including cattle, pigs, sheep, goats, chicken, ostrich, duck, horse, pangolin, elephant calf, buffalo, dolphin, migratory birds, and non-human primates [22–26, 59–70].

The transmission dynamics of *E. fergusonii* in domestic animals are not yet fully understood, but evidence suggests that both direct and indirect routes may play a role. Fecal-oral transmission through contaminated feed, water, or environmental sources is likely a significant mode of spread within and between animal facilities [22, 23, 25, 32, 67, 71]. Additionally, the potential for *E. fergusonii* to be carried asymptomatically by animals and subsequently transmitted to other hosts is a concern, as it may complicate disease recognition and control efforts [22, 23, 61, 72].

The clinical manifestations associated with *E. fergusonii* infection in domestic animals vary widely, ranging from asymptomatic carriage to severe disease. *E. fergusonii* has been associated with a range of clinical manifestations, such as diarrhea, enteritis and septicemia, mastitis, pneumonia, fibrino-necrotic typhlitis, and skin infection [24, 59, 60, 62, 63, 65, 66, 73, 74].

In cattle, *E. fergusonii* has been mostly linked to cases of diarrhea, and mastitis underscoring its potential to cause significant economic losses in dairy and beef production [73, 74]. There are few reports available that implicated *E. fergusonii* as the cause of bovine mastitis [73, 74]. The actual significance of this emerging pathogen as a cause of economically important diseases like mastitis in dairy herds needs more attention in future research. However, the full extent of the clinical impact of *E. fergusonii* in domestic animals remains to be elucidated, and further research is needed to clarify its disease-causing capabilities and potential zoonotic risks.

Several case studies have documented the detrimental impact of *E. fergusonii* on the health and productivity of domestic animals. Few studies reported this emerging pathogen from cases of diarrhea in ruminants. For example, one of the first available reports in diseased animals documented *E. fergusonii* from sheep with symptoms that were initially indistinguishable from Salmonella infection [69]. More recently, this organism was isolated from a lamb suffering from profuse diarrhea on a farm where other animals were febrile and dehydrated, with some mortality. The authors suggested that *E. fergusonii* could be considered the causative agent as other bacterial pathogens like *Salmonella* was not isolated [75]. Also, *E. fergusonii* was isolated from a 4-year-old goat with symptoms of diarrhea and weight loss; after euthanasia, the same bacteria were isolated from various organs like the intestine, lung, liver, and kidney, which shows the systemic dissemination of the causative agent in the host [59]. Another study in Germany described the isolation of *E. fergusonii* from a horse with symptoms of diarrhea and septicemia, highlighting the potential role of this pathogen in gastrointestinal diseases in equine [63]. Years ago, Herráez et al. investigated intestinal lesions, blood, liver, and spleen of two adult ostriches with Fibrino-Necrotic Typhlitis and severe hemorrhagic diarrhea and reported the presence of *E. fergosunii* for the first time in ostrich [62]. The authors of this chapter have also recently documented the fecal carriage of *E. fergusonii* in almost 10% of diseased ostrich chicks suffering from clinical conditions like diarrhea and weight loss [76]. All these reports together suggest that *E. fergusonii* must be considered in the differential diagnosis of bacterial enteric infection and septicemia in farm animals, particularly in small ruminants and ratites. Also, there is one report from the United States, in which *E. fergusonii* was isolated in pure culture from a pneumonic adult cow [60]. The ability of *E. fergusonii* to infect various organ systems, as demonstrated in the goat and horse case reports, raises concerns about its potential for systemic dissemination within the host. Although *E. fergusonii* has been frequently isolated from healthy pigs in different studies, the significance of the health of swine is not clear [64, 77, 78]. Additionally, based on the available literature, no official report is available on the occurrence of *E. fergusonii* in companion animals like dogs and cats. Overall, the prevalence of *E. fergusonii* in domestic animals appears to be underestimated, as it is often misidentified or overlooked.

Escherichia fergusonii has also been reported in wildlife species, which necessitates further research on the pathogenic potential of this emerging pathogen in wildlife and zoonotic risk for humans. For instance, a study by Shah et al. described the isolation of *E. fergusonii* from blood, saliva, and intestine of migratory birds with a rate of 126 out of 183 (69%) samples [22]. Additionally, a case report conducted by Mahato et al. reported *E. fergusonii* from fecal samples in an elephant calf with diarrhea and debility symptoms [65], and another case report in China demonstrated *E. fergusonii* in pangolin with an abdominal skin infection [66]. Also, Glover et al. reported *E. fergusonii* in 23 of 300 (7.66%) non-human primates (vervets and baboons) fecal samples in South Africa [67]. Also, *E. fergusonii* has been isolated in one out of 13 sampled Buffalos [68]. In conclusion, all reports show the wide distribution of this emerging pathogen in wildlife with the possibility of causing disease in some species that require more research.

Apart from the available reports of animals with clinical conditions, many studies have also reported the prevalence of *E. fergusonii* in asymptomatic carrier animals. For instance, a study conducted in South Korea found that *E. fergusonii* was isolated from 23.4% of healthy chickens [61]. Similarly, a survey in Canada identified *E. fergusonii* in 245 of 580 (42.24%) broiler chickens cloacal and cecal samples [23]. Moreover, in another study, *E. fergusonii* was isolated from diverse sources including chicken (11.67%), duck (7.41%), and pigs (7.07%) [25]. Another investigation depicts the prevalence of 18.88% detected *E. fergusonii* among 286 samples of cecal contents or cloacal swabs from chickens and ducks [26]. Wang et al. also isolated *E. fergusonii* in nasal swab samples of pigs (6/250) in China [64]. These findings suggest that *E. fergusonii* is not confined to a single host species and may be more widespread in domestic animal populations than previously recognized. Although the pathogenic potential is not clear from the presented research here, such animal species as chickens, ducks, and pigs should be considered reservoirs of this emerging pathogen that have epidemiological significance [23, 25, 26, 61]. When comparing the prevalence rates across these studies, the available data suggests that poultry and free-living birds may have the highest rate of *E. fergusonii* carriage [22, 23].

In conclusion, the epidemiology of *Escherichia* species, particularly *E. fergusonii*, in domestic and wild animals warrants further investigation. The available evidence suggests that this emerging pathogen may be more prevalent than previously thought, with the potential to cause significant disease in livestock. Ongoing surveillance, improved diagnostic techniques, and a better understanding of the transmission dynamics and pathogenicity of *E. fergusonii* are crucial for mitigating its impact on animal health and addressing potential zoonotic risks. Furthermore, the misidentification of *E. fergusonii* as other gram-negative *Enterobacterales* species in routine culture-based methods highlights the importance of accurate species-level identification for appropriate diagnosis and treatment.

4.2 *Escherichia albertii*

Escherichia albertii has emerged as an important *Escherichia* species with a growing presence in domestic animal populations and human clinical cases worldwide. This bacterium, first isolated from a wild bird in 2003 [40], has since been detected in a variety of domestic animal species, as well as in human diarrheal cases.

E. albertii has been isolated from a diverse range of animal species, including poultries and migratory birds, as well as other mammals such as pigs, dogs, cats, penguins, raccoons, bats, and seals [35, 79–87]. Although the isolation rate varied in different studies, poultry and birds showed the highest overall occurrence; therefore poultry products and contacting birds could potentially act as a potential source for *E. albertii* infections [79–81, 88–90]. Noticeably, in a recent survey conducted in Switzerland, 23.7% of weaning pigs across 24 different farms carried *E. albertii* in their feces that poses swine as a potential reservoir of this emerging pathogen [91]. Another work isolated 12 *E. albertii* out of 270 cloacal specimens from broilers in the USA [81].

This emerging pathogen has been frequently reported in wildlife species worldwide. A report that isolated *E. albertii* from dead Finches in the United States and Scotland incriminates the bacterium as a possible pathogen in wild or captive birds [79]. Surveys conducted in Australia have revealed a considerable prevalence of *E. albertii* in certain bird populations, with 14.3–18% of magpies and 6.7–33% of chickens testing positive [85]. Interestingly, the same studies did not detect the presence of *E. albertii* in other cold-blooded animals like fish, snakes, lizards, crocodiles, and frogs over 10 years [85]. Recently, prevalence studies have reported the isolation of *E. albertii* in wild birds in 5 out of 156 from the cloacal swab with and without clinical symptoms in Japan [92], 31 out of 280 (11.1%) from fecal samples in Switzerland [93] and 9 out of 58 (29.0%) from a cloacal swab in Korea [82].

A recent survey in Okayama prefecture in Japan isolated *E. albertii* from various free-living mammals and birds including martens, foxes, rabbits, safeguard dogs and cats, crows, and starling [87]. Hinenoya et al. investigated 430 rectal samples of raccoons and detected a significant number of 248 (57.7%) *E. albertii* in Japan [84]. Moreover, Ooka et al. have found 26 *E. alberti* strains which consist of 14, and 11 isolates in humans and birds and one strain in a cat [35]. Prevalence of *E. albertii* in a study conducted in Australia has been 0.95% in 945 birds [85]. In addition, Grillová et al. have reported *E. albertii* in three seals and one penguin in the Czech Republic [86]. The identification of *E. albertii* in raccoons, bats, seals, and wild birds suggests that these wild animal populations, particularly birds, may serve as reservoirs for this pathogen.

The occurrence of *E. albertii* in apparently healthy animals raises the possibility of the existence of carrier states, where animals can harbor the pathogen without exhibiting overt clinical signs [82, 83, 92]. This scenario could complicate the diagnosis and understanding of the full clinical presentation of *E. albertii* infections in both animals and humans. Additionally, the heterogeneous nature of *E. albertii* isolates from both animal and human sources suggests that all strains of this pathogen may have zoonotic potential, posing a significant public health concern. Based on the available literature, the pathogenic potential of *E.albertii* is not well-documented in animals, and further research is necessary to elucidate the actual impact on domestic animals' reproduction and health.

4.3 *Escherichia marmotae*

The emergence of *Escherichia marmotae*, as a newly discovered *Escherichia* species, has raised significant concerns regarding its implications for animal and public health. *E. marmotae* was first isolated from fresh fecal samples of seven healthy marmots (*Marmota himalayana*) in China [41] and has since been reported in a variety of domestic and wild animal species, including cattle, avian, migratory birds, wild rodents, wild boars, alpine marmot, and clams (*Venus gallina*) [1, 39, 94–101].

Studies have revealed that the prevalence of *E. marmotae* can be substantial in animal populations. A study in Italy investigated the prevalence of *E. marmotae* in wild boars haunted in Sardina (Italy) and detected 6/61 (9.8%) *E. marmotae* isolates [95]. Similarly, a recent investigation in Belgium that evaluated 38 terrestrial zoo mammals found that *E. marmotae* was present in an alpine marmot examined [99]. Ocejo et al. reported *E. marmotae* in a fecal sample of beef cattle in Northern Spain [94]. Another study revealed the prevalence of 37.2% *E. marmotae* in European starlings [96]. Tawfik et al. isolated *E. marmotae* from a cow rumen sample [97]. Another recent work depicts the presence of *E. marmotae* in the lungs of a healthy wild rodent (mice) in Russia [98], and Sakaguchi et al. reported *E. marmotae* from fecal samples of two urban crows in Japan [100]. Additionally, *E. marmotae* was detected in clams in Italy [101].

These findings suggest that *E. marmotae* has successfully established itself as a plausible emerging pathogen in various animal species, with the potential to cause significant economic and health impacts. Additionally, *E. marmotae* has been detected in environmental samples, such as soil and water, indicating the potential for indirect transmission [1, 39].

The impact of *E. marmotae* on animal health and production cannot be overstated. Moreover, the zoonotic potential of *E. marmotae* raises concerns about its possible transmission to humans, underscoring the need for a comprehensive understanding of its epidemiology and the development of effective prevention and control strategies [102]. **Figure 1** represents the animal reservoirs reported for. Emerging Escherichia species in domestic and farm animals.

4.4 *Escherichia ruysiae*

Another novel *Escherichia* species, *Escherichia ruysiae*, has been described for the first time in association to travelers' diarrhea in a human patient returning from Asian countries [3]. Recent studies have shed light on the prevalence and epidemiology of *E. ruysiae* in livestock and companion animal populations that might have significant implications for the health and well-being of domestic animals.

According to the recent research by Siddi et al., *E. ruysiae* has been detected in one out of 61 (1.6%) haunted wild boars in Italy [95]. Another survey of 500 *Escherichia* isolates from environmental sources in New Zealand found 4 *E. ruysiae* isolates from avian feces [1]. Additionally, Sakaguchi et al. detected one *E. ruysiae* stain from fecal samples of urban crows in Japan [100]. Moreover, an investigation in Switzerland studied 71 *E. ruysiae* strains from 16 countries, mainly from the United States and the United Kingdom (44, 15, and 12 strains isolated from animals, the environment, and humans, respectively). In this study, animal hosts have consisted of companion animals, wild animals, livestock, and poultries [103]. And Leoni et al. isolated one *E.*

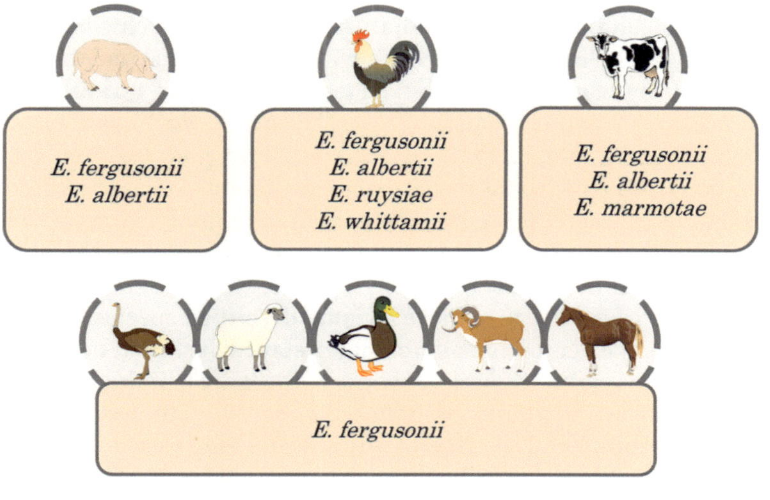

Figure 1.
Prominent domestic farm animal reservoirs reported for the emerging Escherichia *species.*

ruysiae strain from clams in Italy [101]. These researches suggest that *E. ruysiae* may be a common inhabitant of the gastrointestinal tracts of many warm-blooded animals.

Although the pathogenic potential of *E. ruysiae* has not been well-documented in domestic animals, the ability of this bacterium to persist in the environment and potentially contaminate agricultural settings and farm animals is a concern that warrants further investigation [39].

Continued research is essential to fully understand the epidemiology, host range, and pathogenic potential of *E. ruysiae* in animals. Surveillance studies, such as the one conducted by Biggs et al. and Cookson et al., will be crucial in mapping the distribution and prevalence of this emerging *Escherichia* species and informing appropriate mitigation strategies to safeguard animal and public health [1, 39].

4.5 *Escherichia whittamii*

In addition to novel *Escherichia* species, another recently described *Escherichia* species that has garnered attention in the scientific community is *Escherichia whittamii*. This bacterium was first isolated from chicken fecal samples in 2021 and was subsequently named after the renowned *E. coli* researcher Thomas S. Whittam [1, 2, 48]. Based on the available literature, the spectrum of clinical manifestations caused by this novel species and its precise prevalence in human and animal populations remain to be elucidated through further epidemiological investigations.

5. Antimicrobial resistance

The emergence of novel *Escherichia* species, such as *E. fergusonii*, *E. albertii*, *E. marmotae*, and *E. ruysiae*, has raised significant concerns regarding their potential for harboring antimicrobial resistance (AMR) genes. These species, which were previously considered uncommon or even rare, have garnered increasing attention due to their ability to cause human and animal infections, often with clinical presentations similar to those associated with the more well-known *E. coli* [3–6, 26, 76].

Escherichia fergusonii has demonstrated high resistance to a range of antibiotics, including penicillin G, ampicillin, amoxicillin-clavulanic, florfenicol, tetracycline, and trimethoprim-sulfamethoxazole, sulfafurazole, erythromycin, ceftiofur, ceftriaxone, streptomycin, colistin [22–26, 59, 60, 64, 66, 67, 76]. The underlying resistance mechanisms in *E. fergusonii* have been linked to the presence of various resistance genes, such as *bla*$^{CTX\text{-}M}$ and *bla*^{TEM}, *bla*^{CMY}, *bla*^{SHV}, *bla*^{OXA}, *bla*^{ACT}, *aadA*, *strA*, *strB*, *dfrA*, *tet (A, B, C, E, M, X4)*, *sul (1, 2,3)*, *aph*, *cmlA*, *erm*, *floR*, *Inu*, *mef*, *qacL*, *qnrsS*, *gyrA*, *mcr-1*, integron1 which confer resistance to different classes of antibiotics such as beta-lactams and trimethoprim, aminoglycoside, streptomycin, tetracyclines, sulfonamide, erythromycin, phenicol, lincosamide, macrolide, quinolone, and colistin, respectively [22, 23, 25–27, 64, 76, 77].

Similarly, *Escherichia albertii*, a more recently described species, has also demonstrated concerning levels of antimicrobial resistance. It should be noted that compared to other emerging *Escherichia* species, there are a limited number of reports available on antimicrobial resistance in *E. albertii*. Stock et al. investigated the natural susceptibility of 21 *E. albertii* and showed they were naturally resistant to tetracycline, penicillin G, oxacillin, and most macrolides. *E. albertii* was naturally sensitive to all b-lactams (except for penicillin G and oxacillin), azithromycin, and fosfomycin [30]. In another report from China using the whole-genome sequencing approach 85.9% of *E. albertii* isolates were predicted to be multidrug-resistant (MDR) with 35.9% harboring genes related to resistance to 10–14 different antimicrobial classes [29]. A recent report comparing the genomic epidemiology of *E. albertii* isolated in Great Britain from humans and birds reported a wide range of antimicrobial resistance genes including bla^{TEM}, bla^{DHA}, *strA*, *strB*, *aadA*, *dfrA*, *inu(FG)*, *marR*, *mphA*, *gyrA*, *parE*, *qnrB*, *qnrS*, *sul(1,2,3)*, *tet(A,B)*, *uhp(A,T)* that confers resistance to beta-lactams, aminoglycosides, trimethoprims, lincosamides, macrolides, quinolones, sulfonamides, tetracyclines, and fosfomycin respectively [28]. The ability of *E. albertii* to acquire and disseminate these resistance determinants poses a significant challenge in the clinical management of infections caused by this emerging pathogen.

Escherichia marmotae, a species closely related to *E. coli*, has also been resistant to a range of antibiotic classes including beta-lactams, tetracyclines, cephalosporins, sulfonamides, trimethoprim (antimetabolites), and aminoglycosides [94, 96, 98, 99]. Research showed *E. marmotae* harboring a wide range of antimicrobial resistance genes such as bla^{KPC}, bla^{SHV}, $bla^{CTX\text{-}M}$, bla^{CMY}, *tet(A)*, *parC*, *parE*, *fosA*, *aph*, *sul2*, *drfA*, and *aadA*. The presence of these resistance genes in *E. marmotae* underscores the potential for this species to contribute to the growing global challenge of antimicrobial resistance [94, 96, 99, 102, 104].

More recently, *Escherichia ruysiae*, a novel *Escherichia* species isolated from human stool samples, has also been observed to exhibit resistance to various antimicrobial agents, including ampicillin, cefotaxime, sulfamethoxazole-trimethoprim, ciprofloxacin, levofloxacin, and norfloxacin [3, 101, 103]. Whole-genome sequencing analyses have revealed the presence of resistance genes, such as bla^{TEM}, bla^{CTX_M}, *dfrA*, *qnrS*, *aph-Ib*, *sul2*, *tet(A)*, *gyrA*, and *mdfA*-like in *E. ruysiae* isolates, highlighting the need for continued vigilance and research into the antimicrobial resistance profiles of this emerging pathogen [3, 103].

The widespread presence of antimicrobial resistance genes across these novel *Escherichia* species presents a significant public health concern. The ability of these species to acquire and disseminate resistance determinants, either through horizontal gene transfer or clonal expansion, can lead to the development of multi-drug-resistant strains that are increasingly challenging to treat. This, in turn, can result in prolonged illnesses, increased morbidity and mortality, and a greater burden on healthcare systems. To address this growing threat, a multifaceted approach is required, focusing on enhanced surveillance, improved diagnostic capabilities, and the development of novel antimicrobial agents and treatment strategies. Collaborative efforts between clinicians, veterinarians, and public health authorities are crucial to mitigate the risks posed by these emerging *Escherichia* species and their antimicrobial resistance profiles.

6. Public health significance of the emerging *Escherichia* species

While *Escherichia coli* remains the most well-known member of the *Escherichia* genus, the discovery and characterization of several newly described *Escherichia* species, including *E. marmotae*, *E. ruysiae*, and *E. whittamii*, have expanded the genus since 2015. Although some species like *E. fergusonii* and *E. albertii* were described years ago (in 1985 and 2003, respectively), our understanding of their pathogenic potential and public health significance has increased significantly in recent years (**Table 1**) [6, 7, 25].

The epidemiology and pathogenicity of these emerging *Escherichia* species have become the primary subject of extensive investigations worldwide, garnering significant attention. Since most of the novel *Escherichia* species have been reported in asymptomatic or diseased domestic animals and wildlife and have also been implicated in human infections, animals and foods could be potential sources of infection and outbreaks in humans. This section will provide a brief overview of reports on these emerging pathogens and their association with human infections. **Figure 2** represents the most prominent clinical manifestations reported in association with novel emerging *Escherichia* species in humans.

Escherichia fergusonii has been linked to numerous human clinical cases, including bacteremia, inflammatory bowel disease, wound infections, hemolytic uremic syndrome (HUS), cystitis, urinary tract infections, osteomyelitis, uveitis, and biliary infections [7–17, 105–108]. The occurrence of these diverse clinical manifestations underscores the versatility and adaptability of this emerging pathogen.

Of particular note is the association between *Escherichia fergusonii* and hemolytic uremic syndrome (HUS) in humans. HUS is a life-threatening condition characterized by the triad of hemolytic anemia, thrombocytopenia, and acute kidney injury. This severe illness has been reported in several case studies involving *Escherichia fergusonii* as the causative agent [11, 12]. The diverse range of clinical presentations associated with *Escherichia fergusonii* highlights the need for improved diagnostic capabilities and increased awareness among healthcare professionals. Accurate identification of this emerging pathogen is crucial for early detection and implementation of appropriate treatment strategies, as misidentification with other *Escherichia* species could delay appropriate care.

Furthermore, the growing concern regarding antimicrobial resistance in *Escherichia fergusonii* adds to the public health challenge. This species has been reported to exhibit resistance to a variety of antibiotics, as some multi-drug-resistant (MDR) or pan-drug-resistant (PDR) strains have been reported [66, 76]. The emergence of multidrug-resistant strains underscores the urgency in developing new

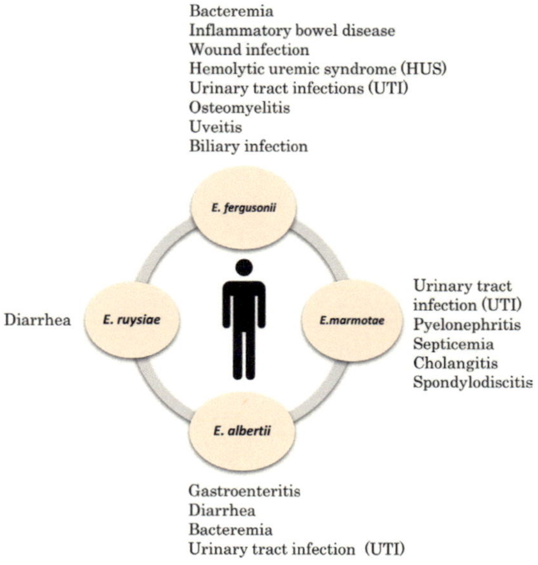

Figure 2.
Prominent clinical manifestations reported in humans in association with emerging Escherichia *species.*

therapeutic options and implementing effective antimicrobial stewardship practices to combat these evolving Escherichia threats.

The clinical manifestations of *E. albertii* infections in humans can range from mild, self-limiting diarrhea to severe, life-threatening complications, such as hemorrhagic colitis, hemolytic uremic syndrome, and even sepsis [6, 109]. Vulnerable populations, including young children, elderly individuals, and immunocompromised patients, are at an increased risk of developing severe disease outcomes [18, 110–112]. For instance, *E. albertii* has been associated with acute diarrhea, gastroenteritis, bacteremia, and urinary tract infection (UTI) [18, 20, 21, 110–114]. Importantly, *Escherichia albertii* has been reported as the cause of six diarrhea outbreaks in Japan in humans between 2003 and 2015 and most of these outbreaks were supposed to be foodborne or waterborne [19]. Another study documented a gastroenteritis outbreak that occurred in 22 patients in Japan, in November 2011 [20].

It is worth noting that some *E. albertii* have reported encoding a potent cytotoxin, Shiga toxin 2 (Stx2a or Stx2f), henceforth has been referred to as Shiga toxin-producing *E. albertii* (STEA) [6, 115–117]. As seen with Shiga toxin-producing *E. coli* (STEC), it is possible that STEA can cause hemorrhagic colitis, hemolytic uremic syndrome (HUS), thrombotic microangiopathy, and renal failure [109, 114, 115]. Furthermore, some strains possess Intimin, an outer membrane attachment protein encoded by the *eae* gene, and therefore can be simply misreported as enteropathogenic *E. coli* (EPEC) [35–38].

The transmission of *E. albertii* is thought to occur primarily through the fecal-oral route, with contaminated food, water, or direct animal-to-human contact serving as potential vectors [6, 19, 21, 35, 114, 117, 118]. Studies have reported the isolation of *E. albertii* from human clinical cases and domestic animal sources, such as poultry, cattle, and companion animals, suggesting the potential for zoonotic transmission [35, 79, 81, 83, 87, 91, 119]. In addition to its ability to cause severe gastrointestinal illness, *E. albertii* has been shown to harbor virulence factors and antimicrobial resistance genes, which can be transmitted to other *Escherichia* species and pose a threat to both animal and human health [28, 29, 37, 38, 117]. This characteristic further emphasizes the need for continued surveillance, improved diagnostic tools, and research into the pathogenic mechanisms of *E. albertii* to mitigate its impact on public and animal health.

While the recent emergence of *Escherichia marmotae* as a possible pathogen in domestic animals, its prevalence and impact on human health are also of growing concern. Recent studies have reported the detection of *E. marmotae* in samples from human patients, particularly in cases of urinary tract infection (UTI) [102, 120]. Furthermore, *E. marmotae* has been reported in four cases, including acute sepsis of unknown origin, postoperative sepsis after cholecystectomy, spondylodiscitis, and upper urinary tract infection [104].

A study by Van Der Putten et al. reported the isolation of *E. ruysiae* from stool samples of human travelers, suggesting that this bacterium may be capable of colonizing the human gut [3]. While the prevalence of *E. ruysiae* in the general human population remains to be thoroughly investigated, detecting this bacterium in travelers raises concerns about its potential for global dissemination. As individuals move between geographical regions, they may act as vectors, carrying and potentially introducing *E. ruysiae* into new environments, where it could then establish itself and threaten both animal and human health [3, 103]. The clinical significance of *E. ruysiae* in humans is an area that requires further research. As this emerging species continues to be recognized, it will be essential to monitor its distribution, identify any associations with human diseases, and develop appropriate prevention and control strategies to mitigate the potential risks it poses to both animal and human populations.

7. Conclusion

The emergence and increasing recognition of novel *Escherichia* species highlight the evolving and multifaceted nature of this important bacterial genus. While *Escherichia coli* remains the best-known and most extensively studied member, the discovery and characterization of species such as *E. fergusonii*, *E. albertii*, *E. marmotae*, *E. ruysiae*, and *E. whittamii* underscore the significant diversification within the *Escherichia* genus.

These emerging *Escherichia* species have demonstrated the potential to pose significant public health and animal health concerns worldwide. Their ability to infect and cause disease in a wide range of hosts, including humans, livestock, pets, and wildlife, raises troubling questions about their zoonotic potential and capacity to cross species barriers. The association of these novel *Escherichia* species with severe gastrointestinal illnesses, such as HUS and diarrhea, further emphasizes the need for improved understanding of their pathogenic mechanisms, virulence factors, and epidemiological profiles.

The growing threat of antimicrobial resistance among these emerging *Escherichia* species, exemplified by the reports of plasmid-mediated colistin resistance in *E. fergusonii*, underscores the urgent need for enhanced diagnostic capabilities, optimized antimicrobial stewardship practices, and the development of new therapeutic options. Effective prevention and control strategies are crucial to mitigate the public health and veterinary risks posed by these evolving *Escherichia* threats.

As the scientific community continues to identify and characterize these novel *Escherichia* species, ongoing research, enhanced surveillance, and collaborative interdisciplinary efforts will be essential to stay ahead of these evolving challenges. Improving our understanding of the taxonomy, genetics, ecology, and pathogenic mechanisms of these bacteria will inform the development of more robust detection methods, comprehensive risk assessment protocols, and targeted intervention strategies. By addressing the multifaceted implications of these emerging *Escherichia* species, the research settings and medical communities can work together to protect both animal and human health in the face of this evolving menace.

Conflict of interest

The authors do not have any conflict of interest to disclose.

Author details

Afagh Torkan and Mahdi Askari Badouei*
Department of Pathobiology, Faculty of Veterinary Medicine, Ferdowsi University of Mashhad, Mashhad, Iran

*Address all correspondence to: askari.m@um.ac.ir

IntechOpen

© 2024 The Author(s). Licensee IntechOpen. This chapter is distributed under the terms of the Creative Commons Attribution License (http://creativecommons.org/licenses/by/4.0), which permits unrestricted use, distribution, and reproduction in any medium, provided the original work is properly cited.

References

[1] Biggs PJ, Moinet M, Rogers LE, Devane M, Muirhead R, Stott R, et al. Draft genome sequences of *Escherichia spp*. isolates from New Zealand environmental sources. Microbiology Resource Announcements. 2024;**13**(3):1-3

[2] Gilroy R, Ravi A, Getino M, Pursley I, Horton D, Alikhan NF, et al. A Genomic Blueprint of the Chicken Gut Microbiome. 2024. DOI: 10.21203/rs.3.rs-56027/v1

[3] BCL VDP, Matamoros S, Mende DR, Scholl ER, Consortium C, Schultsz C. *Escherichia ruysiae sp*. nov., a novel gram-stain-negative bacterium, isolated from a faecal sample of an international traveller. International Journal of Systematic and Evolutionary Microbiology. 2021;**71**(2):1-7. Available from: http://www.ncbi.nlm.nih.gov/pubmed/33406029

[4] Yu D, Banting G, Neumann NF. A review of the taxonomy, genetics, and biology of the genus *Escherichia* and the type species *Escherichia coli*. Canadian Journal of Microbiology. 2021;**67**(8):553-571

[5] Gaastra W, Kusters JG, van Duijkeren E, LJA L. *Escherichia fergusonii*. In: Veterinary Microbiology. Vol. 172. 2014. pp. 7-12

[6] Muchaamba F, Barmettler K, Treier A, Houf K, Stephan R. Microbiology and epidemiology of *Escherichia albertii*—An emerging elusive foodborne pathogen. Microorganisms. 2022;**10**(5):875. Available from: https://www.mdpi.com/2076-2607/10/5/875/htm

[7] Zang YM, Liu JF, Li G, Zhao M, Min YG, Ping ZZ, et al. The first case of *Escherichia fergusonii* with biofilm in China and literature review. BMC Infectious Diseases. 2023;**23**(1):1-7

[8] Gokhale VV, Therese KL, Bagyalakshmi R, Biswas J. Detection of *Escherichia fergusonii* by PCR-based DNA sequencing in a case of delayed-onset chronic endophthalmitis after cataract surgery. Journal of Cataract and Refractive Surgery. 2014;**40**(2):327-330. Available from: https://journals.lww.com/jcrs/fulltext/2014/02000/detection_ofescherichia_fergusoniiby_pcr_based_dna.22.aspx

[9] Lagacé-Wiens PRS, Baudry PJ, Pang P, Hammond G. First description of an extended-spectrum-β-lactamase-producing multidrug-resistant *Escherichia fergusonii* strain in a patient with cystitis. Journal of Clinical Microbiology. 2010;**48**(6):2301-2302

[10] Savini V, Catavitello C, Talia M, Manna A, Pompetti F, Favaro M, et al. Multidrug-resistant *Escherichia fergusonii*: A case of acute cystitis. Journal of Clinical Microbiology. 2008;**46**(4):1551-1552

[11] Baek SD, Chun C, Hong KS. Hemolytic uremic syndrome caused by *Escherichia fergusonii* infection. Kidney Research and Clinical Practice. 2019;**38**:253-255

[12] Hwang S, Chang HH, Bae S, Kim YK, Kim J. A case of resembling hemolytic uremic syndrome caused by *Escherichia fergusonii* in an immunocompetent adult. Chonnam Medical Journal. 2022;**58**(1):64

[13] Adesina T, Nwinyi O, De N, Akinnola O, Omonigbehin E. First detection of carbapenem-resistant *Escherichia fergusonii* strains harbouring beta-lactamase genes from clinical samples. Pathogens. 2019;**8**(4):1-13

[14] Beli E, Duraku E. *Escherichia fergusonii* strains isolated from clinical specimens in Albania. Journal of Multidisciplinary Engineering Science and Technology (JMEST). 2017;**4**:7085-7088. Available from: www.jmest.org

[15] Dahal RH, Choi YJ, Kim S, Kim J. Differentiation of *Escherichia fergusonii* and *Escherichia coli* isolated from patients with inflammatory bowel disease/ ischemic colitis and their antimicrobial susceptibility patterns. Antibiotics. 2023;**12**(1):1-14

[16] Jiang YY, Zhang Y, Hu Y, Guo Y. *Escherichia fergusonii* bacteremia after esophagectomy: A case report and literature review. Journal of International Medical Research. 2023;**51**(4):1-6

[17] Vanegas-Rodríguez ÉS, López-Jácome LE, Becerra-Lobato N, Colín-Castro CA, Franco-Cendejas R. *Escherichia fergusonii* in a patient with a traumatic amputation of the right pelvic limb. Cirugia y Cirujanos (English Edition). 2020;**88**(91):51-53

[18] Iguchi A, Takemura T, Ogura Y, Nguyen TTH, Kikuchi T, Okuno M, et al. Genomic characterization of endemic diarrheagenic *Escherichia coli* and *Escherichia albertii* from infants with diarrhea in Vietnam. PLoS Neglected Tropical Diseases. 2023;**17**(4):1-13

[19] Masuda K, Ooka T, Akita H, Hiratsuka T, Takao S, Fukada M, et al. Epidemiological aspects of *Escherichia albertii* outbreaks in Japan and genetic characteristics of the causative pathogen. Foodborne Pathogens and Disease. 2020;**17**(2):144-150

[20] Konno T, Yatsuyanagi J, Takahashi S, Kumagai Y, Wada E, Chiba M, et al. Isolation and identification of *Escherichia albertii* from a patient in an outbreak of gastroenteritis. Japanese Journal of Infectious Diseases. 2012;**65**:203-207. Available from: http://blast.ddbj.nig.ac.jp/top-j.html

[21] Ooka T, Tokuoka E, Furukawa M, Nagamura T, Ogura Y, Arisawa K, et al. Human gastroenteritis outbreak associated with *Escherichia albertii*, Japan. Emerging Infectious Diseases. 2013;**19**(1):144-146

[22] Shah A, Alam S, Kabir M, Fazal S, Khurshid A, Iqbal A, et al. Migratory birds as the vehicle of transmission of multi drug resistant extended spectrum β lactamase producing *Escherichia fergusonii*, an emerging zoonotic pathogen. Saudi Journal of Biological Sciences. 2022;**29**(5):3167-3176

[23] Simmons K, Islam MR, Rempel H, Block G, Topp E, Diarra MS. Antimicrobial resistance of *Escherichia fergusonii* isolated from broiler chickens. Journal of Food Protection. 2016;**79**(6):929-938

[24] Parin U, Kirkan S, Arslan SS, Yuksel HT. Molecular identification and antimicrobial resistance of *Escherichia fergusonii* and *Escherichia coli* from dairy cattle with diarrhoea. Veterinary Medicine Journal. 2018;**63**(3):110-116

[25] Tang B, Chang J, Chen Y, Lin J, Xiao X, Xia X, et al. *Escherichia fergusonii*, an Underrated Repository for Antimicrobial Resistance in Food Animals. 2022. Available from: https://journals.asm.org/journal/spectrum

[26] Lin J, Tang B, Zheng X, Chang J, Ma J, He Y, et al. Emergence of Incl2 plasmid-mediated colistin resistance in avian *Escherichia fergusonii*. FEMS Microbiology Letters. 2022;**369**(1):1-9

[27] Liu R, Xu H, Guo X, Liu S, Qiao J, Ge H, et al. Genomic characterization of two *Escherichia fergusonii* isolates

harboring mcr-1 gene from farm environment. Frontiers in Cellular and Infection Microbiology. 2022;**12**:1-11

[28] Bengtsson RJ, Baker KS, Cunningham AA, Greig DR, John SK, Macgregor SK, et al. The genomic epidemiology of *Escherichia albertii* infecting humans and birds in Great Britain. Nature Communications. 2023;**14**(1):1-13. Available from: https://www.nature.com/articles/s41467-023-37312-3

[29] Luo L, Wang H, Payne MJ, Liang C, Bai L, Zheng H, et al. Comparative genomics of Chinese and international isolates of *Escherichia albertii*: Population structure and evolution of virulence and antimicrobial resistance. Microbial Genomics. 2021;**7**(12):000710. Available from: https://www.microbiologyresearch.org/content/journal/mgen/10.1099/mgen.0.000710

[30] Stock I, Rahman M, Sherwood KJ, Wiedemann B. Natural antimicrobial susceptibility patterns and biochemical identification of *Escherichia albertii* and hafnia alvei strains. Diagnostic Microbiology and Infectious Disease. 2005;**51**(3):151-163

[31] Gangiredla J, Mammel MK, Barnaba TJ, Tartera C, Gebru ST, Patel IR, et al. Draft genome sequences of *Escherichia albertii*, *Escherichia fergusonii*, and strains belonging to six cryptic lineages of *Escherichia spp*. Genome Announcements. 2018;**6**(18):1-2

[32] Maheux AF, Boudreau DK, Bergeron MG, Rodriguez MJ. Characterization of *Escherichia fergusonii* and *Escherichia albertii* isolated from water. Journal of Applied Microbiology. 2014;**117**(2):597-609

[33] Lindsey RL, Garcia-Toledo L, Fasulo D, Gladney LM, Strockbine N. Multiplex polymerase chain reaction for identification of *Escherichia coli*, *Escherichia albertii* and *Escherichia fergusonii*. Journal of Microbiological Methods. 2017;**140**:1-4

[34] Dadvar A, Tabar GH, Badouei MA, Nemati A, Farsiani H. An improved multiplex-polymerase chain reaction method for simultaneous identification and discrimination of emerging *Escherichia* and *Shigella* species. International Journal of Enteric Pathogens. 2023;**11**(4):128-133. Available from: https://enterpathog.abzums.ac.ir/Article/ijep-5621

[35] Ooka T, Seto K, Kawano K, Kobayashi H, Etoh Y, Ichihara S, et al. Clinical significance of *Escherichia albertii*. Emerging Infectious Diseases. 2012;**18**(3):488-492

[36] Hyma KE, Lacher DW, Nelson AM, Bumbaugh AC, Janda JM, Strockbine NA, et al. Evolutionary genetics of a new pathogenic *Escherichia* species: *Escherichia albertii* and related *Shigella boydii* strains. Journal of Bacteriology. 2005;**187**(2):619-628

[37] Nimri LF. *Escherichia albertii*, a newly emerging enteric pathogen with poorly defined properties. Diagnostic Microbiology and Infectious Disease. 2013;**77**(2):91-95

[38] Bhatt S, Egan M, Critelli B, Kouse A, Kalman D, Upreti C. The evasive enemy: Insights into the virulence and epidemiology of the emerging attaching and effacing pathogen *Escherichia albertii*. Infection and Immunity. 2019;**87**(1):1-32

[39] Cookson AL, Marshall JC, Biggs PJ, Rogers LE, Collis RM, Devane M, et al. Whole-genome sequencing and virulome analysis of *Escherichia coli* isolated from New Zealand environments of contrasting observed land use. Applied

and Environmental Microbiology. 2022;**88**(9):1-19

[40] Huys G, Cnockaert M, Janda JM, Swings J. *Escherichia albertii sp*. nov., A diarrhoeagenic species isolated from stool specimens of Bangladeshi children. International Journal of Systematic and Evolutionary Microbiology. 2003;**53**(3):807-810

[41] Liu S, Jin D, Lan R, Wang Y, Meng Q, Dai H, et al. *Escherichia marmotae* sp. nov., isolated from faeces of Marmota himalayana. International Journal of Systematic and Evolutionary Microbiology. 2015;**65**(7):2130-2134

[42] Castellani A, Chalmers A. Manual of Tropical Medicine. 3rd ed. New York: Williams Wood and Co.; 1919

[43] Clermont O, Christenson JK, Denamur E, Gordon DM. The clermont *Escherichia coli* phylo-typing method revisited: Improvement of specificity and detection of new phylo-groups. Environmental Microbiology Reports. 2013;**5**(1):58-65

[44] Clermont O, Gordon DM, Brisse S, Walk ST, Denamur E. Characterization of the cryptic *Escherichia* lineages: Rapid identification and prevalence. Environmental Microbiology. 2011;**13**(9):2468-2477

[45] Clermont O, Dixit OVA, Vangchhia B, Condamine B, Dion S, Bridier-Nahmias A, et al. Characterization and rapid identification of phylogroup G in *Escherichia coli*, a lineage with high virulence and antibiotic resistance potential. Environmental Microbiology. 2019;**21**(8):3107-3117

[46] Farmer JJ, Fanning GR, Davis BR, O'hara CM, Riddle C, Hickman-Brenner FW, et al. *Escherichia fergusonii* and Enterobacter taylorae, two new species of enterobacteriaceae isolated from clinical specimens. Journal of Clinical Microbiology. 1985:77-81

[47] Okuno M, Arimizu Y, Miyahara S, Wakabayashi Y, Gotoh Y, Yoshino S, et al. *Escherichia* cryptic clade I is an emerging source of human intestinal pathogens. BMC Biology. 2023;**21**(1):1-16

[48] Pallen MJ. Valid publication of names for bacterial species from the chicken gut. International Journal of Systematic and Evolutionary Microbiology. 2024;**74**(7):006445. Available from: https://www.microbiologyresearch.org/content/journal/ijsem/10.1099/ijsem.0.006445

[49] Brenner DJ, Davis BR, Steigerwalt AG, Riddle CF, McWhorter AC, Allen SD, et al. Atypical biogroups of *Escherichia coli* found in clinical specimens and description of *Escherichia hermannii sp*. nov. Journal of Clinical Microbiology. 1982;**15**(4):703-713. Available from: https://journals.asm.org/doi/10.1128/jcm.15.4.703-713.1982

[50] Hata H, Natori T, Mizuno T, Kanazawa I, Eldesouky I, Hayashi M, et al. Phylogeneticsoffamilyenterobacteriaceae and proposal to reclassify *Escherichia hermannii* and *Salmonella subterranea* as Atlantibacter hermannii and Atlantibacter subterranea gen. Nov., comb. nov. Microbiology and Immunology. 2016;**60**(5):303-311. Available from: https://onlinelibrary.wiley.com/doi/full/10.1111/1348-0421.12374

[51] Brenner DJ, McWhorter AC, Knutson KL, Steigerwalt AG. *Escherichia vulneris*: A new species of enterobacteriaceae associated with human wounds. Journal of Clinical Microbiology. 1982;**15**(6):1133-1140. Available from: https://journals.asm.org/doi/10.1128/jcm.15.6.1133-1140.1982

[52] Alnajar S, Gupta RS. Phylogenomics and comparative genomic studies delineate six main clades within the family enterobacteriaceae and support the reclassification of several polyphyletic members of the family. Infection, Genetics and Evolution. 2017;**54**:108-127

[53] Burgess NRH, McDermott SN, Whiting J. Aerobic bacteria occurring in the hind-gut of the cockroach, Blatta orientalis. Epidemiology and Infection. 1973;**71**(1):1-8. Available from: https://www.cambridge.org/core/journals/epidemiology-and-infection/article/aerobic-bacteria-occurring-in-the-hindgut-of-the-cockroach-blatta-orientalis/D0F87B596A4DDE73CD01F7C97519B3D3

[54] Priest FG, Barker M. Gram-negative bacteria associated with brewery yeasts: Reclassification of Obesumbacterium proteus biogroup 2 as Shimwellia pseudoproteus gen. Nov., sp. nov., and transfer of *Escherichia* blattae to Shimwellia blattae comb. nov. International Journal of Systematic and Evolutionary Microbiology. 2010;**60**(4):828-833. Available from: https://www.microbiologyresearch.org/content/journal/ijsem/10.1099/ijs.0.013458-0

[55] Tamura K, Sakazaki R, Kosako Y, Yoshizaki E. Leclercia adecarboxylata Gen. Nov., Comb. Nov., formerly known as *Escherichia adecarboxylata*. Current Microbiology. 1986;**13**(4):179-184 Available from: https://link.springer.com/article/10.1007/BF01568943

[56] Touchon M, Perrin A, De Sousa JAM, Vangchhia B, Burn S, O'Brien CL, et al. Phylogenetic background and habitat drive the genetic diversification of *Escherichia coli*. PLoS Genetics. 2020;**16**(6):e1008866. Available from: https://journals.plos.org/plosgenetics/article?id=10.1371/journal.pgen.1008866

[57] Walk ST, Alm EW, Gordon DM, Ram JL, Toranzos GA, Tiedje JM, et al. Cryptic lineages of the genus *Escherichia*. Applied and Environmental Microbiology. 2009;**75**(20):6534-6544

[58] Walk ST. The 'cryptic' *Escherichia*. EcoSal Plus. 2015;**6**(2)

[59] Hariharan H, López A, Conboy G, Coles M, Muirhead T. Isolation of Escherichia fergusonii from the feces and internal organs of a goat with diarrhea. Canadian Veterinary Journal. 2007;**48**(6):630-631

[60] Rimoldi GM, Moeller RB. *Escherichia fergusonii* associated with pneumonia in a beef cow. Journal of Veterinary Medicine. 2013;**2013**:1-3

[61] Oh JY, Kang MS, An BK, Shin EG, Kim MJ, Kwon JH, et al. Isolation and epidemiological characterization of heat-labile enterotoxin-producing *Escherichia fergusonii* from healthy chickens. Veterinary Microbiology. 2012;**160**(1-2):170-175

[62] Herráez P, Rodríguez AF, De Los E, Monteros A, Acosta AB, Jaber JR, et al. Fibrino-necrotic typhlitis caused by *Escherichia fergusonii* in ostriches (*Struthio camelus*). Avian Diseases. 2005;**49**(1):167-169

[63] Weiss ATA, Lübke-Becker A, Krenz M, van der Grinten E. Enteritis and Septicemia in a horse associated with infection by *Escherichia fergusonii*. Journal of Equine Veterinary Science. 2011;**31**(7):361-364

[64] Wang J, Wan X, Meng H, Olsen RH, Chen X, Li L. Efflux pumps and different genetic contexts of tet(X4) contribute to high tigecycline resistance in *Escherichia fergusonii* from pigs. International Journal of Molecular Sciences. 2023;**24**(8):1-10

[65] Mahato G, Dutta M, Sarma KK, Arif SA, Gogoi SM, Basumatary P, et al. First report of isolation of Enteropathogenic *Escherichia fergusonii* from the faeces of Elephantcalf (*Elephas Maximus*). Exploratory Animal and Medical Research. 2023;**13**(2):178-183

[66] An F, Wang K, Wei S, Yan H, Xu X, Xu J, et al. First case report of pustules associated with *Escherichia fergusonii* in the chinese pangolin (Manis pentadactyla aurita). BMC Veterinary Research. 2023;**19**(1):1-7

[67] Glover B, Wentzel J, Jenkins A, Van Vuuren M. The first report of *Escherichia fergusonii* isolated from non-human primates, in Africa. One Health. 2017;**3**:70-75

[68] Kabali E, Pandey GS, Munyeme M, Kapila P, Mukubesa AN, Ndebe J, et al. Identification of *Escherichia coli* and related enterobacteriaceae and examination of their phenotypic antimicrobial resistance patterns: A pilot study at a wildlife-livestock interface in Lusaka, Zambia. Antibiotics. 2021;**10**(3):1-17

[69] Bain M, Green C. Isolation of Escherichia fergusonii in cases clinically suggestive of salmonellosis. Veterinary Records. 1999;**144**:511

[70] Rios EA, Santos J, García-Meniño I, Flament-Simon SC, Blanco J, García-López ML, et al. Characterisation, antimicrobial resistance and diversity of atypical EPEC and STEC isolated from cow's milk, cheese and dairy cattle farm environments. LWT. 2019;**108**:319-325

[71] Busayo O, Oluyege JO, Famurewa O, Oluwaseun OA, Olowe BM, Oluyege JO, et al. Molecular identification of Escherichia coli and new emerging enteropathogen, *Escherichia fergusonii*, from drinking water sources in Ado-Ekiti, Ekiti state, Nigeria. Journal of Microbiology Research (Rosemead, CA). 2017;**2017**(3):45-54. Available from: https://www.researchgate.net/publication/323599844

[72] Savini V, Catavitello C, Bianco A, Masciarelli G, Astolfi D, Balbinot A, et al. First Enteric *Escherichia fergusonii* from Italy. Infez Med. 2009;**17**(4):259-260

[73] Jahan NA, Godden SM, Royster E, Schoenfuss TC, Gebhart C, Timmerman J, et al. Evaluation of the matrix-assisted laser desorption ionization time of flight mass spectrometry (MALDI-TOF MS) system in the detection of mastitis pathogens from bovine milk samples. Journal of Microbiological Methods. 2021;**182**:1-8

[74] Al-Haddadi W, Elshafie A, Al-Ansari A, Al-Mawly J, Al-Hatali R, Al-Habsi H, et al. Bovine mastitis in Oman is mainly associated with environmental bacteria that show high resistance to commonly used antibiotics. Archives of Microbiology and Immunology. 2020;**04**(02):38-50

[75] Kirkpatrick MA, Timms LL, Kersting KW, Kinyon JM. Case report: Jejunal Hemorrhage syndrome of dairy cattle. Bov Pract (Stillwater). 2001;**35**(2):104-116. Available from: https://bovine-ojs-tamu.tdl.org/bovine/article/view/1640

[76] Torkan A, Badouei MA. Investigating the virulence-associated genes and antimicrobial resistance of *Escherichia fergusonii* isolated from diseased ostrich chicks. Comparative Immunology, Microbiology and Infectious Diseases. 2024;**112**:102226. Available from: https://linkinghub.elsevier.com/retrieve/pii/S0147957124001036

[77] Kakita T, Shigemura H, Fukuda A, Katamune C, Nidaira M, Kudeken T, et al.

Antimicrobial resistance and molecular epidemiological analysis of *Escherichia fergusonii* harboring the mcr gene in pigs and broiler chickens in Okinawa, Japan. Journal of Veterinary Medical Science. 2023;**85**(2):149-156. Available from: https://www.ncbi.nlm.nih.gov/pmc/journals/2350/

[78] Rayamajhi N, Bin CS, Shin SW, Jung BY, Lim SK, Yoo HS. Plasmid typing and resistance profiling of *Escherichia fergusonii* and other enterobacteriaceae isolates from south Korean farm animals. Applied and Environmental Microbiology. 2011;**77**(9):3163-3166

[79] Oaks JL, Besser TE, Walk ST, Gordon DM, Beckmen KB, Burek KA, et al. *Escherichia albertii* in wild and domestic birds. Emerging Infectious Diseases. 2010;**16**(4):638-646

[80] Hinenoya A, Li XP, Zeng X, Sahin O, Moxley RA, Logue CM, et al. Isolation and characterization of *Escherichia albertii* in poultry at the pre-harvest level. Zoonoses and Public Health. 2021;**68**(3):213-225

[81] Wang H, Zhang L, Cao L, Zeng X, Gillespie B, Lin J. Isolation and characterization of *Escherichia albertii* originated from the broiler farms in Mississippi and Alabama. Veterinary Microbiology. 2022;**267**:109379

[82] Oh JY, Kang MS, Hwang HT, An BK, Kwon JH, Kwon YK. Epidemiological investigation of eaeA-positive *Escherichia coli* and *Escherichia albertii* strains isolated from healthy wild birds. Journal of Microbiology. 2011;**49**(5):747-752

[83] Hinenoya A, Shima K, Asakura M, Nishimura K, Tsukamoto T, Ooka T, et al. Molecular Characterization of Cytolethal Distending Toxin Gene-Positive *Escherichia coli* from Healthy Cattle and Swine in Nara, Japan. 2014. Available from: http://www.biomedcentral.com/1471-2180/14/97

[84] Hinenoya A, Nagano K, Awasthi SP, Hatanaka N, Yamasaki S. Prevalence of *Escherichia albertii* in raccoons (Procyon lotor), Japan. Emerging Infectious Diseases. 2020;**26**(6):1304. Available from: /pmc/articles/PMC7258444/

[85] Gordon DM. Reservoirs of Infection: The Epidemiological Characteristics of an Emerging Pathogen *Escherichia albertii*. Australian National University, Canberra. Available from: https://www.agriculture.gov.au/sites/default/files/sitecollectiondocuments/animal-plant/emergency/wildlifeexoticdiseaseprogram/08-09/epidemiological-char-pathogen-albertii.pdf [Accessed: Sep 2024]

[86] Grillová L, Sedláček I, Páchníková G, Staňková E, Švec P, Holochová P, et al. Characterization of four *Escherichia albertii* isolates collected from animals living in Antarctica and Patagonia. Journal of Veterinary Medical Science. 2018;**80**(1):138-146

[87] Naka A, Hinenoya A, Awasthi SP, Yamasaki S. Isolation and characterization of *Escherichia albertii* from wild and safeguarded animals in Okayama prefecture and its prefectural borders, Japan. Journal of Veterinary Medical Science. 2022;**84**(9):1299-1306

[88] Asoshima N, Matsuda M, Shigemura K, Honda M, Yoshida H, Oda T, et al. Isolation of *Escherichia albertii* from raw chicken liver in Fukuoka City, Japan. Japanese Journal of Infectious Diseases. 2015;**68**(3): 248-250

[89] Maeda E, Murakami K, Sera N, Ito K, Fujimoto S. Detection of *Escherichia albertii* from chicken meat and giblets.

Journal of Veterinary Medical Science. 2015;**77**(7):871-873

[90] Wang H, Li Q, Bai X, Xu Y, Zhao A, Sun H, et al. Prevalence of eae-positive, lactose non-fermenting *Escherichia albertii* from retail raw meat in China. Epidemiology and Infection. 2016;**144**(1):45-52. Available from: https://www.cambridge.org/core/journals/epidemiology-and-infection/article/prevalence-of-eaepositive-lactose-nonfermenting-escherichia-albertii-from-retail-raw-meat-in-china/FDE5C297F656AFDD62EA2BB4276540FD

[91] Barmettler K, Biggel M, Treier A, Muchaamba F, Stephan R. Livestock as possible reservoir of *Escherichia albertii* in Switzerland. Schweizer Archiv für Tierheilkunde. 2023;**165**(5):299-306

[92] Hinenoya A, Awasthi SP, Yasuda N, Nagano K, Hassan J, Takehira K, et al. Detection, isolation, and molecular characterization of *Escherichia albertii* from wild birds in West Japan. Japanese Journal of Infectious Diseases. 2022;**75**(2):156-163

[93] Barmettler K, Biggel M, Treier A, Muchaamba F, Vogler BR, Stephan R. Occurrence and characteristics of *Escherichia albertii* in wild birds and poultry flocks in Switzerland. Microorganisms. 2022;**10**(11):299-306

[94] Ocejo M, Tello M, Oporto B, Lavín JL, Hurtado A. Draft genome sequence of *Escherichia* marmotae E690, isolated from beef cattle. Microbiology Resource Announcements. 2020;**9**(32):1-3

[95] Piras F, Gymoese P, Torpdahl M, Meloni MP, Cuccu M, Migoni M, et al. Pathogenic Profile and Antimicrobial Resistance of *Escherichia coli*, *Escherichia Marmotae* and *Escherichia* 2 Ruysiae Detected from Hunted Wild Boars in Sardinia 3 4 Giuliana Siddi. 2024. Available from: https://ssrn.com/abstract=4782812

[96] Souguir M, Châtre P, Drapeau A, François P, Azaiez S, Ncir S, et al. Molecular characterization of highly prevalent *Escherichia coli* and *Escherichia marmotae* resistant to extended-spectrum cephalosporins in European starlings (*Sturnus vulgaris*) in Tunisia. Microbiology Spectrum. 2023;**11**(5):1-12

[97] Tawfik MA, Aboseidah AA, Heneidak S, Rasmey AHM. Kinetic study of biohydrogen production improvement via dark fermentation of sugarcane molasses by *Escherichia marmotae*. Egyptian Journal of Botany. 2023;**63**(2):551-561

[98] Zhurilov PA, Andriyanov PA, Tutrina AI, Razheva IV, Liskova EA, Gladkova NA, et al. Characterization and comparative analysis of the *Escherichia marmotae* M-12 isolate from bank vole (Myodes glareolus). Scientific Reports. 2023;**13**(1):1-12

[99] De Witte C, Vereecke N, Theuns S, De Ruyck C, Vercammen F, Bouts T, et al. Presence of broad-spectrum beta-lactamase-producing enterobacteriaceae in zoo mammals. Microorganisms. 2021;**9**(4):1-15

[100] Sakaguchi K, Tanabe M, Takizawa S, Kasahara S, Denda T, Koide S, et al. Zoonotic potential and antimicrobial resistance of *Escherichia spp*. in urban crows in Japan-first detection of E. Marmotae and E. Ruysiae. Comparative Immunology, Microbiology and Infectious Diseases. 2023;**100**:102040

[101] Leoni F, Sacchini L, Pieralisi S, Angelico G, Magistrali CF, Cucco L, et al. Occurrence and temporal distribution

of extended-spectrum β-lactamase-producing *Escherichia coli* in clams from the central Adriatic, Italy. Frontiers in Microbiology. 2023;**14**:1219008

[102] Sinha T, Merlino J, Rizzo S, Gatley A, Siarakas S, Gray T. Unrecognised: Isolation of *Escherichia marmotae* from clinical urine sample, phenotypically similar to *Escherichia coli*. Pathology. 2024;**56**(4):577-578

[103] Campos-Madueno EI, Aldeia C, Sendi P, Endimiani A. *Escherichia ruysiae* may serve as a reservoir of antibiotic resistance genes across multiple settings and regions. Microbiology Spectrum. 2023;**11**(4):1-8

[104] Sivertsen A, Dyrhovden R, Tellevik MG, Bruvold TS, Nybakken E, Skutlaberg DH, et al. *Escherichia marmotae*—A human pathogen easily misidentified as *Escherichia coli*. Microbiology Spectrum. 2022;**10**(2):1-8

[105] Freney J, Gavini F, Ploton C, Leclerc H, Fleurette J. Isolation of *Escherichia fergosonii* from a patient with septicemia in France. European Journal of Clinical Microbiology. 1987;**6**(1):78. Available from: https://link.springer.com/article/10.1007/BF02097203

[106] Bours PHA, Polak R, Hoepelman AIM, Delgado E, Jarquin A, Matute AJ. Increasing resistance in community-acquired urinary tract infections in Latin America, five years after the implementation of national therapeutic guidelines. International Journal of Infectious Diseases. 2010;**14**(9):e770-e774

[107] Funke G, Hany A, Altwegg M. Isolation of *Escherichia fergusonii* from four different sites in a patient with pancreatic carcinoma and cholangiosepsis. Journal of Clinical Microbiology. 1993;**31**:2201-2203

[108] Lai CC, Cheng A, Huang YT, Chung KP, Lee MR, Liao CH, et al. *Escherichia fergusonii* bacteremia in a diabetic patient with pancreatic cancer. Journal of Clinical Microbiology. 2011;**49**(11):4001-4002

[109] Ooka T, Ogura Y, Katsura K, Seto K, Kobayashi H, Kawano K, et al. Defining the genome features of *Escherichia albertii*, an emerging enteropathogen closely related to *Escherichia coli*. Genome Biology and Evolution. 2015;**7**(12):3170-3179

[110] Zaki MES, Eid AE, El-Kazzaz SS, El-Sabbagh AM. Molecular study of *Escherichia albertii* in pediatric urinary tract infections. The Open Microbiology Journal. 2022;**15**(1):139-144

[111] Hinenoya A, Yasuda N, Hibino T, Shima A, Nagita A, Tsukamoto T, et al. Isolation and characterization of an *Escherichia albertii* strain producing three different toxins from a child with diarrhea. Japanese Journal of Infectious Diseases. 2017;**70**(3):252-257

[112] Liu Q, Wang H, Zhang S, Yan G, Yang X, Bai X, et al. *Escherichia albertii* isolated from the bloodstream of a patient with liver cirrhosis in China: A case report. Heliyon. 2023;**9**(11):1-4

[113] Fujioka M, Yoshioka S, Ito M, Ahsan CR. Characterization of the emerging enteropathogen *Escherichia Albertii* isolated from urine samples of patients attending sapporo area hospitals, Japan. International Journal of Microbiology. 2022;**2022**:1-6

[114] Murakami K, Etoh Y, Tanaka E, Ichihara S, Horikawa K, Kawano K, et al. Shiga toxin 2f-producing *Escherichia*

albertii from a symptomatic human. Japanese Journal of Infectious Diseases. 2014;**67**:204-208. Available from: http://homepage.usask.ca/

[115] Ori EL, Takagi EH, Andrade TS, Miguel BT, Cergole-Novella MC, Guth BEC, et al. Diarrhoeagenic *Escherichia coli* and *Escherichia albertii* in Brazil: Pathotypes and serotypes over a 6-year period of surveillance. Epidemiology and Infection. 2019;**147**:1-9

[116] Brandal LT, Tunsjø HS, Ranheim TE, Løbersli I, Lange H, Wester AL. Shiga toxin 2a in *Escherichia albertii*. Journal of Clinical Microbiology. 2015;**53**:1454-1455

[117] Gomes TAT, Ooka T, Hernandes RT, Yamamoto D, Hayashi T. *Escherichia albertii* pathogenesis. EcoSal Plus. 2020;**9**:1

[118] Hirose S, Konishi N, Sato M, Suzumura K, Obata H, Ohtsuka K, et al. Growth and survival of *Escherichia albertii* in food and environmental water at various temperatures. Journal of Food Protection. 2024;**87**(4):1-7

[119] Leszczyńska K, Święcicka I, Daniluk T, Lebensztejn D, Chmielewska-Deptuła S, Leszczyńska D, et al. *Escherichia albertii* as a potential enteropathogen in the light of epidemiological and genomic studies. Genes (Basel). 2023;**14**(7):1-19

[120] Katrodiya N, Patel N, Patel S, Adedayo Animasaun D, Oyedeji S, Rajani P, et al. Isolation and identification of brevibacillus and *Escherichia spp*. from urinary tract of infected patients. Annals of Biology. 2022;**38**(1):134-147